250 different from low-fat slow cooker recipes

breakfast, lunch and dinner recipes
Healthy diet

Compiled by David C. Kellogg

250 different from low-fat slow cooker recipes

Albondigas 1

Alpine Chicken 1
America's Favorite Pot Roast 2

Apple butter 2
Apples 'N Port 2
Bread and apple pudding 3
Arizona Chuck Wagon Beans 3

Rice With Chicken 4
Chicken and beans with Asian spices 4
Fall Vegetable Minestrone 5
BBQ 5 beef sandwiches

Barbecue beef sandwiches 5

Grilled pork 6

Chicken with basil 6

Chicken stew with Basque 6

Beef And Broccoli 7

Beef and pasta 7

Beef stew 8

Boeuf Stroganoff 8

Beef tips in mushroom sauce 9

Bloody Mary Chicken 9

Burger Heaven Casserole 9

Chicken Crockpot Busy Day and Rice 10
Chou Burger Bake 10

Cabbage soup 10
Cafe Chicken 11
California Vegetable Cheese Cooking 11

Poulet et riz Campbell's One Dish 11

Caccitore Chicken Cheats 12

Cheddar fondue 12
Cherry Cobbler 13

Chicken and pasta with cheese and artichokes 13
Chicken simmered with cheese 13
Chicken and macaroni with mushrooms 14
Chicken and rice 14

Chicken A La King 14
Chicken and stuffing 15
Brunswick Chicken Stew 15
Casablanca Chicken 15

Chicken Cordon Bleu 16
Chicken dinner in a slow cooker 16
Chicken in mushroom sauce 16
Chicken Italiano 17

Chicken and noodle soup 17
Chicken and noodle soup - 2 18
Chicken Paella 18
Parmesan chicken 19

Chicken stew 19
Poulet Stroganoff 20
Stroganoff au poulet #2 20
Poulet Stroganoff Supreme 20

Chicken soup with vegetables 21

Chicken and vegetable chowds 21
Chicken wings in barbecue sauce 22

Chicken wings in honey sauce 22

Chicken wings in teriyaki sauce 22
Chicken with Lima beans C / P 23
Chile 23
Chili Mac Pot 23

Chili Pasta Bake 24
Chinese beef and pea pods 24
Beef stew and Chinese vegetables) 24
Chops in a slow cooker 25

Chop Suey on rice 25
Beef and pork chili in pieces 26
Chicken with cola 26
Colorful chicken stew 26

Chili comforting Crock Pot) 27

Rooster with Wine 27
Scallops, ham and potato 28
Salted beef hash 28
Country Captain Chicken with Rice 28

Cowboy Stew 29
Cozy Crock Comfort Serves-6 29
Creamy chicken and wild rice 30

Creamy red potatoes 30

Creamy red potatoes and chicken 30

Potted pineapple chicken 31

Crockpot Apple Pie 31

Haricots au four Crockpot 31

Beef and peppers Crockpot 32

Boeuf et bouillon Crockpot 32

Beef stew crockpot) 33

Crockpot Beef with Mushrooms and Red Wine Sauce 33

Crockpot Big Bowl of Red Chili 33

Soupe aux haricots noirs Crockpot 34

Breakfast Crockpot 34

Poulet Crockpot 35

Chicken Crock Pot - 2 35

Poulet Crockpot & Farce 35
Crockpot Chicken Chili 35

Fajitas au poulet Crockpot 36

Chicken Marengo Crock Pot 36
Crockpot Chicken Paprika 36

Soupe de tortilla au poulet Crockpot 37
Soupe de Tortilla au Poulet Crockpot # 2 37
Crock-Pot Chili 38
Crockpot 38 colorful chicken stew

Casserole de poulet Crockpot Company 39
Fettuccine crémeuse au poulet Crockpot 39
Crockpot Easy French Dip Sandwiches 40
Crockpot Family Favorite Pot Roast 40

Crockpot 41 Green Chili Chicken Stew
Jambon Crockpot et haricots de Lima 41
Crockpot 41 homemade turkey dinner
Poulet Italien Crockpot 42

Poulet Italien Crockpot # 2 42
Crockpot Lemon Chicken 42
Crockpot 43 Meatloaf Recipe
Crockpot Mexican Pork 43

Crockpot Multi-Bean Soup 44
Crockpot 44 pork chop dinner
Crockpot Potato Chowthed 45
Crockpot 45 pulled pork fajitas

Chicken and salted vegetables Crockpot 45

Crockpot Soup 46
Crock Pot Soup - 1 46

Chicken salsa with Crockpot sour cream 47

Crockpot 47 Broken Pea Soup
Crockpot Swiss Steak 47
Crockpot Tuscan Pasta 48
CrockPot Vegetable Pasta 48

Cuban black beans 49
Crock Pot simplest chicken 49
Easy baked beans 50
Easy Cassoulet 50

Easy Hearty Turkey Chili 50
Easy Italian vegetable soup 51
Eight-layer casserole 51
Favorite Family Chile 52

Forgotten Minestrone 52

Frankfurters avec macaroni et fromage 52
Roast pork with garlic 53
Shiny pork chops 53
Ginger Pork Wraps 54

Ham and potatoes with gratin 54
Hamburger and noodle soup 54
Baked ham 55

Hearty dinner made with Italian spaghetti 55

Hearty meatballs 56

Herb turkey and wild rice casserole 56

Herb turkey breast 56

Hot Crab Dip 57

Gâteau Crockpot Hot Fudge 57

Hot Texas Chili Soup 57

Hungarian Goulash 58

Italian beef and green pepper sandwiches 58

Dinner Knot Italian Butterfly 59

Italian Roast 59

Italian spaghetti sauce 59

Italian tortellini stew 60

Italian Turkey Rice Dinner 60

Italian Turkey Dinner 61

Jambalaya 61

Fajitas to prepare 62

Filling 62
Tortillas 62

Toppings 62
Mom Chicken Stew 62
Mexi Dip 63
Mexican Green Chile 63

Mom's homemade chicken soup 63
Roast chuck with onion and mustard leaf 64
Chicken casserole without a look 64
Poire Streusel 64

Beijing pork chops 65
Hot Chicken Sandwich Peles 65

Pepper steak in pot 66
Pepsi and pork in slow cooker 66

Pineapple Chicken 66
Pioneer Beans 66
Polynesian steak strips 67
Pork-spice meatballs with tomato sauce 67

Pork and black bean chili) 68
Dinner pork chops 68
Pork chops stuffed with cornbread with jalapeno and pecans 68
Pork chops and potatoes with mustard sauce 69

Pizza Pot 69

Pot Roast 70
Potato and leek chowds 70

Potato and mushroom chowds 70

Red beans and rice 71
Fried beans 71
Rustic vegetable soup 71
Chicken Salsa 72

Sausage pasta stew 72
Dinner of sausages and sauerkraut 72
Fajitas with salted beef 73
Salted pot

Dumplings

1/2 pound ground chuck 1/2
onion - chopped
2 garlic cloves, chopped
1/4 cup instant rice and 1 uncooked
egg
Salt and pepper - to taste
4 ounces chopped green peppers - canned, drained
1 grated carrot
14 1/2 ounces simmered tomatoes - canned
4 cups hot water
2 cups low-fat beef stock -- or water
1 teaspoon dried oregano
2 tablespoons chopped fresh parsley or coriander

In a bowl, combine beef, onion, garlic, rice, egg, salt and pepper to taste. Form into 1 1/2-inch meatballs. Place the grated peppers and carrots in the bottom of the slow cooker. Pour the tomatoes evenly over the top. Place meatballs on top of tomatoes. Pour into water, broth, oregano and parsley or coriander. Cover and cook on LOW 5 1/2 to 6 hours. Garnish this popular Mexican soup with sprigs of fresh coriander or mint, and serve with flour tortillas.

Per serving: 121 Calories); (kcal); 7g total fat; 7g protein; 9g carbohydrates; 45mg Cholesterol; 48mg sodium

Alpine chicken

6 portions

2 teaspoons chicken broth granules
1 tablespoon chopped fresh parsley 3/4
teaspoon poultry seasoning
4 ounces diced Canadian bacon
2 carrots -- minced,--(up to 3) 1 rib celery -
- thinly sliced ,- (up to 2) 1 small onion --
thinly sliced
1/4 cup water
6 chicken breast halves, boneless skinless
1 can of condensed cheddar cheese soup -- (11 oz))
1 tablespoon all-purpose flour
2 tablespoons sliced chilli
2 tablespoons grated Parmesan cheese
1 packet of large egg noodles - cooked, drained (16 - oz)

In a small bowl, combine broth granules, chopped parsley and poultry seasoning; Set aside. Layer in a slow cooker, in order. Bacon, carrots, celery and Canadian onions. Add water. Remove skin, if desired, and excess fat from chicken; rinse and dry. Put the meat in a slow cooker. Sprinkle with half of the reserved seasoning mixture. Garnish with remaining chicken and sprinkle with remaining seasoning mixture. Mix soup and flour; spoon on top. DO NOT STIR.

Cover and cook over high heat for 3 to 3 and a half hours or low for 6-8 hours or until chicken is tender and chicken juices are clean and vegetables are tender. Spread cooked noodles in a 2-1/2-quarter shallow grill-proof serving quartdish. Arrange chicken over noodles. Mix soup mixture and vegetables until smooth. Pour the vegetables and some of the liquid over the chicken. Sprinkle with chilli and Parmesan cheese. 6. Grill 6 inches of heat source for 6-8 minutes or until lightly browned.

America's Favorite Pot Roast

3 1/2 pounds roasted tip sirloin, adorned
with 1/4 cup flour
2 teaspoons salt 1/8
teaspoon pepper
3 carrots -- ,, peeled and sliced
3 potatoes -- peeled and quartered
2 small onions, sliced
1 stem celery -- cut into 2" pieces
1 2 Oz Jar mushrooms - drained or 1/4 cup mushroom sauce 3
tablespoons flour
1/4 cup water

Cut off any excess fat from the roast; brown and drain if you use chuck or another heavily marbled cut. Mix 1/4 cup flour, salt and pepper. Coat the meat with the flour mixture. Place all vegetables except mushrooms in Crock-Pot and garnish with roast (roast cut in half, if necessary, to fit easily). Spread the mushrooms evenly on top of the roast. Cover and cook over low heat for 10 to 12 hours. If desired, turn to High for the last hour to soften the vegetables and make a sauce. To thicken the sauce, make a smooth paste of 3 tablespoons of flour and water and stir in Crock-Pot. Season to taste before serving. Serves 4 to 6

Apple butter

Makes 4 cups

12 med. Granny Smith or other cooking apples, peeled and cut into fourth 1 1/2 cups
packaged brown sugar
1/2 cup apple juice
1 tsp ground spices
1 tsp ground nutmeg 1/2
teaspoon ground cloves

Mix all ingredients in a slow cooker of 5 to 6 qt. Cover and cook on LOW 8-10 hours. or until the apples are very tender. Crush apples with potato pestle or large fork. Cook uncovered on LOW 1 to 2 hours, stirring occasionally, until very thick. Cool for about 2 hours. Pour the apple butter into a container. Cover and refrigerate for up to 3 weeks.
By tbs. cal 30, 0g fat, 0g sat fat, sat 0mg chol, 0mg turf, carb 9g, 1g fibre, prot 0g

Apples 'N Port

4 whole cooking apples -- (4 to 6) 1/2
tbsp raisins or currants
1 tbsp brown sugar
1/4 tsp nutmeg
1/4 tbsp ground cinnamon
2/3 tst. port wine

Basic apples and cut a score around the sides about 1/3 down from the top. Fill the score with raisins or currants, and garnish with brown sugar, lightly pressing the sugar towards the centre of the fruit. Place the apples at the bottom of the slow cooker and pour the port over them, seeing that some go into each apple center. Cover and cook low for 3 to 4 hours, or until apples are tender. Serve with excess port sauce poured over apples. Serves 4 to 6.

Note: These apples are excellent hot or cold, and especially well served with rich vanilla ice cream or whipped cream.

Per serving: 225 calories; fat trace; 1 g protein; 51g carbohydrates; 3g dietary fiber; 0mg Cholesterol; 12mg sodium.

Apple pie bread pudding

12 slices of reduced-calorie white bread - torn into medium-sized pieces 3 1/2
cups cooking apples -- cored, peeled and chopped
1 cup unsweetened apple juice 1/2
cup lemon-lime soda
Appropriate sugar substitute for cooking on equal 1/2 cup sugar 1
1/2 teaspoons apple pie spices

Spray the slow cooker with a butter-flavoured non-stick spray. Mix the bread pieces and apples in a slow cooker. In a small bowl, combine apple juice, soda, sugar substitute and apple pie spice. Drizzle evenly over the bread mixture. Mix gently to mix. Cover and cook for 6 hours over low heat or until cooked. Mix well before serving.

Serves six. Each serving   equals: 157 cal; 1 g fat; 5 g pro; 32 g carbo;233 mg sodium; 2 g fiber.

Arizona Chuck Cart Beans

1 pound of sea beans - Dried or Pinto
6 cups water
1/4 Pound pork loins, lean, boneless - diced 1
large onion - chopped
1 clove garlic -- finely chopped
1 large green pepper -- chopped
1 1/2 Pounds Round Steak - cubed
1 1/2 teaspoons salt
1/2 teaspoon oregano -- crumbled 1/4
teaspoon red pepper
1/4 teaspoon ground cumin 8
Ounces tomato sauce

Pick up the beans and rinse well. Mix the beans and water in a large kettle. Bring to a boil; cover; cook for 2 minutes. Remove from heat and let stand for 1 hour, then pour into slow cooker. Brown salted pork in a large frying pan; remove with a slotted spoon for the stove; sauté onion, garlic and green pepper in pan drips; remove with a slotted spoon for the stove. Brown beef, a few pieces at a time in pan drips; casserole; remove from the stove with a slotted spoon; stir in salt, oregano, red pepper, cumin and tomato sauce. Add more water, if necessary to bring the liquid level over the beans. Cook over low heat for 10 hours or over high heat for 6 hours, or until beans are tender.

Calories 391.7 fat 11.9 fibers 14.8

Pollo rice with Pollo chicken

1/2 teaspoon Salt
1/4 C. Pepper
1 clove garlic - crushed
1 Tsp. Oregano
2 Tsp. Chili Powder
8 skinless chicken thighs 1/2 C
chicken broth
2 Tbs. Vin
Red 1 10 Oz Peas, frozen -- thawed 2 C
rice, cooked
2 Tbs. Cilantro -- freshly chopped

In a small bowl, combine salt, pepper, garlic, oregano and chili powder. Sprinkle the spice mixture on both sides of the chicken pieces. Put the chicken in a slow cooker. Pour broth and wine over chicken. Cover and cook over low heat for 5 to 6 hours. Remove chicken and cover to keep warm. Turn the control to the height. Add the peas. Cover and cook over high heat for 7 to 10 minutes. Stir in cooked rice and chicken until smooth. Sprinkle with coriander and serve.

Per serving; 358 Calories; 6g fat (16.6% calories from fat); 34g protein; 38g carbohydrates; 4g dietary fibre; 115mg cholesterol; 581mg sodium. 4 servings

Asian spicy chicken and beans

1/2 cup dry packaged sea beans or 1(15 ounces) can bean, rinsed and drained. 1/2 cup dry packaged red beans or 1(15 ounces) can red beans, rinsed and drained.
1 pound boneless skinless chicken breasts, cut into half-inch cubes. 3 large
carrots, sliced diagonally
2 to 3 teaspoons chopped garlic, to taste
2 to 3 teaspoons chopped ginger root or 1 to 2 teaspoons ground ginger, to taste 1 (14 1/2
ounces) can reduce-sodium fat-free chicken broth
2 tablespoons cornstarch
1/2 teaspoon crushed red pepper
2 to 3 tablespoons reduced sodium soy sauce
4 cups cooked rice
Sliced and high green onions, to garnish
chopped peanuts to garnish

If using dried beans, place dry beans in a large saucepan and cover with 2-inch water; boiling heat; boil, uncovered for 2 to 3 minutes. Remove from heat, cover and set aside for at least 1 hour and up to 4 hours. Drain the soaked water and rinse the beans. Place canned beans, chicken, carrots, garlic, ginger and 1 1/4 cups chicken stock in a slow cooker; stir well. Cover and cook over low heat until beans are tender for about 5 and a half to 6 hours.

Turn the slow cooker high. Mix the cornstarch with the rest of the broth of one-and-a-half cup and add to the mixture in the stove; stir in crushed red pepper. Cover and cook until thickened, about 30 minutes. Stir in soy sauce. Serve over rice; sprinkle with green onions and peanuts.

Makes 6 servings, about 1 1/2 cups each.
Per serving: Calories: 375 Fat: 3g Fibre: 10g Carbohydrates: 56g Sodium: 285mg Protein: 30g Chol:46mg

Minestrone with autumn vegetables

2 14.5 oz   vegetable stock in cans
1 18 oz   undrained crushed tomatoes
3 medium carrots -- chopped (1 1/2 cups)
3 small zucchini -- cut into one- and two-inch slices
1 medium yellow pepper -- cut into 1/2-inch pieces 8 medium green onions -- sliced (1/2 cup)
2 garlic cloves -- finely chopped
2 cups shredded cabbage
2 teaspoons dried marjoram
1 teaspoon salt
1/4 teaspoon pepper
1 cup raw instant rice 1/4 cup chopped fresh basil

Mix all ingredients except rice and basil in a slow 3 1/2 to 6 litre cooker. Cover and cook over low heat for 6 to 8 hours or until vegetables are tender. Stir in rice. Cover and cook over low heat for about 15 minutes or until rice is tender.

Per serving: 195 Calories); (kcal); 2g total fat; 7g protein; 39g carbohydrates; 1mg cholesterol; 1198 mg sodium

BBQ beef sandwiches

2 1/2 lbs lean boneless chuck roasts
1/4 cup tomato ketchup
1 tablespoon Dijon-style mustard
2 tablespoons brown sugar
1 clove garlic - crushed
1 tablespoon Worcestershire sauce
2 tablespoons red wine vinegar
1/4 teaspoon liquid smoke flavouring
1/4 teaspoon salt
1/8 teaspoon pepper
10 French buns or sandwiches -- (10 to 12)

Put the beef in a slow cooker. Mix the rest of the ingredients, except the rolls. Pour over the meat. Cover and cook on LOW 8 to 9 hours. Refrigerate or make sandwiches now. Shred beef pulling it apart with 2 forks. Add a cup of sauce. Heat the mixture in the microwave or on the stovetop. Pour over hot, open-faced buns or buns. Garnish with extra hot sauce if desired.

For 10-12 servings: 298 calories; 16g fat; 18g protein; 19g carbohydrates; 1g dietary fibre; 55mg cholesterol; 373mg sodium.

Barbecue beef sandwiches

3 pounds roasted beef boneless chuck
1 cup barbecue sauce 1/2
cup canned apricot
2 tablespoons red or green pepper- chopped
1 tablespoon Dijon mustard
2 teaspoons brown sugar - packaged
1 small onion - sliced
12 whole hamburger buns or Kaiser rolls - split

Remove excess fat from beef. Cut the beef into 4 pieces. Place beef in a 4- or 5-litre slow cooker. Mix the rest of the ingredients except the buns; pour over the beef. Cover and cook over low heat for 7 to 8 hours or until beef is tender. Remove beef from slow cooker. Cut beef into thin slices; stir in sauce again. Cover and cook over low heat for another 20 to 30 minutes or until beef is hot. Fill buns with beef mixture.

Per serving (1 sandwich): cals 410; fat 16 g; chol 70 mg; sodium 520 mg; carbohydrates 39 g, fiber 2 g; protein 29 g

Spread the buns with horseradish sauce for a delicious kick of flavor!

Grilled pork:

Makes 8 servings

2 lbs boneless pork loin
1 tst chopped onion
3/4 tst.
3/4 tbsp barbecue sauce

Mix all ingredients in a slow cooker. Cook covered for 5-6 hours or until meat is very tender. Drain and slice or shred the pork. I serve it on wheat loaves.

Chicken with basil

4 whole skinless chicken breasts 1/2
teaspoon pepper
1/2 teaspoon basil
1 can of celery soup cream
1/2 whole green pepper - sliced

Put the chicken breasts in a slow cooker. Sprinkle with pepper and basil. Spread soup over chicken. Arrange the slices of green pepper on top of the soup. Cover and cook over low heat for 6 to 8 hours.

Per serving: 287 calories; 4g fat; 55g protein; 3g carbohydrates; 1g dietary fibre; 141mg Cholesterol; 391mg sodium.

Basque-style chicken stew

2 tablespoons olive oil
6 slices of turkey bacon, Louis Rich -- diced 1/2 inch 8
ounces of mushroom -- sliced
1 green pepper - cubed 1"
1 red pepper - cubed 1"
1 bunch of green onions - 1/2 - 1" chunks
1 pound boneless skinless chicken breasts - 1" cubes
2 tablespoons balsamic vinegar 1/2
teaspoon marjoram
1/2 teaspoon salt 1/4
teaspoon pepper
1/4 cup fat-free chick. broth, 1/3 less turf., Swan -- see note 2 cups
tomatoes, canned -- 16 oz

Heat the olive oil in a large frying pan; fry the bacon until golden brown. Add mushrooms, peppers and green onions and sauté for one minute. Add vinegar and cook for another minute, scraping the golden pieces from the bottom of the pan. Book. Put the chicken in a slow cooker. Add the sautéed bacon and vegetable mixture to the pan, the olives (optional). Mix remaining ingredients in a bowl and mix. Pour over chicken and vegetables in slow cooker. Cover and cook over low heat for 8 to 10 hours. Can be served on rice.

The recipe called for skinless chicken breast halves and regular chicken broth. (You get more meat if you use boneless, skinless chicken breasts.
Serving size (1/4 recipe) Per serving: 203 Calories, 8.7 g fat, 2.4 g fibre

Beef and broccoli

1 pound boneless beef steak -- cut fat, cubed 1 4.5-ounce green giant jar® sliced
mushrooms - drained
1 medium onion -- quartered 1/2 cup
condensed beef stock
3 tablespoons bought tériyaki baste and icing
1 tablespoon sesame seeds
1 teaspoon dark sesame oil - if desired
2/3 cup regular white rice with uncooked long grains
1 1/3 cups water
2 tablespoons water
1 tablespoon cornstarch
2 cups select green giant® 100% frozen broccoli florets

In a slow cooker of 3 1/2 to 4 quarters, combine beef, mushrooms, onion, broth, bast and teriyaki icing, sesame seeds and sesame oil; mix well. Cover; cook at low setting for 8 to 10 hours. About 35 minutes before serving, cook the rice in 1 1/3 cups of water as indicated on the package. Meanwhile, in a small bowl, combine 2 tablespoons of water and cornstarch; maïs; mix well. Stir cornstarch mixture and broccoli into beef mixture. Cover; cook at low setting for an additional 30 minutes or until broccoli is tender. Serve over rice.

Makes 4 servings (1 1/4 cups). Calories.350. Fat.6 g. Carbs.37 g. Protein.30 g. Sodium... 600 mg... Fiber... Threeg.

Beef and pasta

Makes 8 servings (1 cup)

2 (14 oz) cans of tomatoes with juice, broken
1 1/2 cups water
1 tsp parsley flakes 1/4
teaspoon garlic powder
1/4 tsp onion powder 1
tsp salt
1/ tsp pepper
1 tsp liquid sauce browning
1 1/2 lbs lean ground beef
8 oz Rotini pasta (less than 4 cups)

Mix the first 8 ingredients in a large bowl. Stir well. Add ground beef. Mix. Turn into 3 1/2 qt. slow cooker. Cover. Cook on LOW for 6 to 8 hours. or HIGH for 3 to 4 hours. Add pasta. Stir. Cook on HIGH for 15 to 20 minutes until tender.

Per serving: 322cal, 13.6 g fat, 584 mg turf, 21 g prot,28 g carbohydrates

Beef stew

Service size: 8

1 pound beef stew - cubed, 1"
8 teaspoons McCormick Beef Stew seasoning -- (1/2 pack)
15 ounces green beans, canned -- 1 can
15 ounces canned black beans -- 1 can (store rite) 15
ounces peas, canned -- 1 can
15 ounces corn, canned -- 1 can
3 cups water

Put in a slow cooker and simmer all day (about 8 hours).

If you can't find McCormick Beef Stew seasoning use another brand of seasoning or use your own favorite spices i.e.:dire: salt, pepper, garlic, or onion soup mix :)

NOTES: Per serving: 309.4 cal, 12.4 g (35.6%) fat, 6.4 g fibre, 646 mg sodium, 27.1 g carbohydrates, 23.5 g protein

Boeuf Stroganoff

1 1/2 lbs beef, dressed - see note
1 onion, chopped
8 oz sliced mushrooms
1 tsp Dijon mustard
2 tsp dried parsley 1/2
teaspoon salt
1/2 teaspoon dill --
dried 1/4 teaspoon
pepper
1 clove garlic - chopped
1/2 tst all-purpose flour -- see note 1 can
fat-free beef broth -- see 3/4 tst of low-
fat gras sour cream
6 tbsp egg noodles, Barilla -- cooked, see note

Cut the fat from the steak. Wrap steak in heavy plastic wrap; freeze for 30 minutes. Unpacked steak; déballé; cut the steak diagonally over the grain into half-inch-thick slices. Place steak, onion and the following 7 ingredients in a 3-quarter electric slow cooker. Combine flour and broth in a bowl; stir with a whisk until mixed.

Add broth mixture to stove; stir well. Cover; cook over low heat for 8 hours or until tender. Turn off the slow cooker; remove the lid. Leave to rest for 10 minutes. Stir in sour cream. Serve stroganoff over noodles.

Notes: Had 1 1/2 lbs of extra lean beef stew in cubes and used it as it was). To compensate for the extra beef, I increased the broth to use the whole box (was 1 cup), and the flour (was 1/3 cup). And, because the extra beef gave me extra portions, I increased the amount of noodles to give me the right nutritional analysis.

Per serving: 436 calories; 8g fat; 38g protein; 53g carbohydrates; 133mg Cholesterol; 409mg sodium

Beef tips in mushroom sauce

2 pounds lean chuck - cut into 1 - 3/4 inches pieces 1
can 98% fat-free cream of mushroom soup
1 pkg. onion soup mix
1 can sugar-free sprite or 7up

Put the meat in the slow cooker. Pour the soup and onion mixture over the meat. Add Sugar Free Sprite/7up. Cook in slow cookery jar all day over low heat (or high for at least 4 hours). Turn off and let stand 30 minutes before serving.

Makes 8 servings.

I added canned sliced mushrooms (drained) and served on rice.

Poulet Bloody Mary

4 whole boneless skinless chicken breasts
33 3/4 ounces Bloody Mary mix (I use extra spicy)

Wash, peel and remove fat from chicken breasts and place in a slow cooker. Pour Bloody Mary mixture over chicken breasts, turn slow cooker to low and cook over low heat for 8 hours.

Per serving: 305 calories; 3g fat; 56g protein; 11g carbohydrates; 2g dietary fibre; 137mg Cholesterol; 1026mg Sodium.

Burger Heaven Casserole

16 oz extra lean beef gr. (or turkey)
2 cups sliced raw potatoes
1 and 1/2 cup sliced carrots (I used frozen)
1 cup chopped celery 1/2
cup chopped onion
1 cup frozen peas - thawed
1 cup frozen and thawed whole corn
1 10 oz can make a tomato soup requested
healthily 1/2 cup water
1 tsp dried parsley flakes
1 can of mushrooms
Salt and pepper

In the large frying pan, brown meat, onion and celery mixture and mushrooms. In the slow cooker container - sprayed with butter-flavoured spray, mix the mixture of meat, potatoes, carrots, peas and corn. stir in tomato soup, water, parsley flakes and salt and pepper to taste. Cover and cook over low heat for 6 to 8 hours.

6 - 1 cup portions
243 calories - 7 fat gm - 17 gm. protein - 28 gm. carbohydrates - 333 mg. Sodium (more if you add extra salt) 33 mg calcium - 4 gm. Fibre.

Busy day crockpot chicken and rice

1 lB boneless skinless chicken breasts
2 cans 98% fat-free cream of chicken soup 1 can
98% fat-free cream ofroni mushroom soup 1 can
rice-a-roni chicken flavor

Put chicken and soups in slow cooker and light at low end for 8-10 hours. When you get home, cook the rice according to the package instructions. Serve chicken and sauce over rice.
Easily Doubles! Per serving: 173 calories; 2g fat; 28g protein; 10g carbohydrates; 1g dietary fibre; 66mg Cholesterol; 317mg sodium.

Chou Burger Bake
Makes 6 servings

1 (1 lb) pkg. (aboutenviron 6 cups) 3/4 cup shredded cabbage and
3/4 lb lean ground beef
1/2 teaspoon salt
1/4 teaspoon ground black
pepper 1 med. onion,finely
chopped 1 cup long grain rice
1 (26 oz) can large spaghetti sauce low in fat 1/2
cup water
1/4 teaspoon dried basil leaves,
crushed 1/4 teaspoon seasoned salt

Place 1/2 of the cabbage and carrots in a 3 1/2 qt slow cooker. Crumble the ground beef on top. Sprinkle with one to 1/4 teaspoon of salt and 1/8 teaspoon of pepper. Divide the onion evenly, then the rice over the whole.

Garnish with remaining cabbage, salt and pepper. Combine spaghetti sauce, water, basil and seasoned salt; pour over the cabbage. Cover and cook on LOW for 5 to 6 hours. or until the rice is tender.
Per serving: cal 358, carb 42g, prot 16g, 14g fat, sat sat 5g fat, chol 42mg, turf 985mg

Cabbage roll soup

1 pound on the round floor
3 1/2 cups water
2 cups coarsely chopped green cabbage
1 cup carrot, sliced 1/2
cup sliced celery
1/2 cup chopped onion
1/2 teaspoon dried dill
1/2 teaspoon dried oregano
1/2 teaspoon dried basil 1/2
teaspoon pepper
3 cans of beef consumed -- undiluted --10.5 ounces per box 2 cans of diced tomatoes --non-14.5 ounces per box 1/2 cup undrained undrained converted rice

Brown meat in a non-stick skillet overmedium-high heat; well flow. Place meat in a 4-quarter electric slow cooker; quarts; incorporate water and the next 10 ingredients. Cover; cook over low heat for 8 hours. Increase heat setting to high; stir in rice. Cover and cook for another 30 minutes or until rice is tender. Yield: 10 servings (serving size: 1 1/3 cups). Per serving: Calories 178; protein 14.9 g; fat 5.8 g; carbohydrates 17.3 g; fiber 2.2 g; cholesterol 46 mg; iron 2.4 mg; sodium 776 mg; calcium 48 mg.

Coffee chicken

2 1/2 Lb skinless chicken breast halves - cut into eighths 1 onion -
chopped
2 garlic -- chopped
Salt and white pepper to taste 1
green pepper - diced
1 Medium tomato - Ripe and peeled -- Seeded and chopped 1 cup
dry white wine
1 Pinch cayenne pepper

Mix all ingredients in a slow cooker. Cover the pot and bring it down. Cook for 6 to 8 hours or until chicken is tender. YIELD: Makes 6 servings

California Vegetable Cheese Cook

4 cups frozen carrots, broccoli and cauliflower mixture, thawed 1/2 cup finely chopped onion (can use frozen chopped onion) 1 (10-3/4 oz) can Healthy Demand Cream of Mushroom Soup 1/4 cup (a 2-ounce jar) chopped pimiento, drained
1-1/2 cup Velveeta Light melted cheese cubes

Spray the slow cooker container with butter-flavoured cooking spray. In a prepared container, combine thawed vegetables and onion. Add mushroom soup, pimiento and cheese. Mix well to combine. Cover and cook on LOW for 4 to 6 hours. Mix well before serving.

140 calories, 3 gm fibers, , 4 fat 13 gm proteins, , 13 gm carbohydrates, , 236 mg sodium, 373 mg calcium gm

Campbell's One Dish Poulet et Riz

1 can of mushroom soup cream - Campbell 98% FF 1 cup
water
3/4 cup white rice, regular -- raw 1/4
teaspoon paprika
1/4 teaspoon pepper
1 teaspoon garlic salt - my own addition
4 chicken breast halves -- peeled and boneless

In a 2 tt shallow baking dish, combine soup, water, rice, paprika and pepper. Place chicken on rice mixture. Sprinkle with extra paprika and pepper. Cover. Bake at 375 degrees for 45 minutes or until chicken and rice are cooked. For creamy rice, increase water to 1 1/3 cups.

PORTIONS: 4

Caccitore Chicken Cheaters

6 skinless, boneless chicken breast halves
1 (28 ounces) potty spaghetti sauce
2 greenpeppers, seeded and cubed
8 ounces fresh mushrooms, sliced
1 onion, diced
2 tablespoons chopped garlic

Put the chicken in the slow cooker. Garnish with spaghetti sauce, green peppers, mushrooms, onion and garlic. Cook over low heat for 7 to 9 hours. Serve!

Yield: 5 servings

Calories 283, Protein 37g, Total Fat 5g, Sodium 742mg, Cholesterol 82mg, Carbohydrates 21g, Fibre 4g

Cheddar Fondue

1/4 cup butter or margarine 1/4
cup all-purpose flour 1/2
teaspoon salt -- optional 1/4
teaspoon pepper
1/4 teaspoon mustard powder
1/4 teaspoon Worcestershire sauce 1
1/2 cups skimmed milk
2 cups grated cheddar cheese
bread cubes, ham cubes, frozen sausages

In a saucepan, melt butter; stir in flour, salt if desired, pepper, mustard and Worcestershire sauce until smooth. Gradually add the milk. Bring to a boil; cook and stir for 2 minutes or until thickened. Reduce heat. Add cheese; cook and stir until melted. Transfer to a fondue pot or slow cooker; keep warm.

Serve with bread, ham, sausages and/or broccoli.

NOTES: Per serving: 165 cal,13.3 g fat, 0 g fiber, 312 mg turf, 4.4 g carbohydrates, 7.2 g protein

Per serving (using 2% milk): 161.1 cal.12.8 g (71.0%) fat, 0g fibre, 313mg grass, 4.5g carbohydrates, 7.2g protein per serving (using 2% milk)

Per serving (using 1% milk): 158.2 cal.12.5 g (70.6%) fat, 0g fibre, 313mg grass, 4.5g carbohydrates, 7.2g protein per serving (using 1% milk)

Per serving (skimmed milk): 155.7 cal.12.1 g (69.9%) fat, 0g fibre, 313mg grass, 4.5g carbohydrates, 7.3g protein per serving using (skimmed milk)

Cobbler Cerise

Makes 6 servings

1 can (21 oz) cherry pie filling
1 cup all-purpose flour
1/4 cup sugar
1/4 cup margarine or butter, melted
1/2 cup milk
1 tsp baking powder 1/2
teaspoon almond extract
1/4 teaspoon salt.

Spray inside 2-3 1/2 qt. Simmer with a cooking spray. Pour the pie filling into the stove. Beat remaining ingredients with spoon until smooth. Spread dough over pie filling. Cover and cook on HIGH 1 1/2 to 2 hours. or until the toothpick inserted in the centre comes out clean.

Per serving: cal 270,fat 8g, fat sat 2g, chol 0mg, turf 330mg, carb 49g, fiber 2g, prot 3g

Chicken and artichoke pasta with cheese

1 lb boneless skinless chicken breasts -- cubed (1 to 1 1/2) 4 oz
roasted red peppers -- chopped (4-6)
15 ounces artichoke hearts - in quarters
8 oz fat-free American cheese
2 teaspoons Worcestershire sauce
1 can 98% fat-free cream of mushroom soup 2
cups fat-free grated cheddar cheese
4 cups hot cooked pasta
with salt and pepper
flavour

In a saucepan of 3 1/2 quarters or more, combine chicken, peppers, artichokes, American cheese, Worcestershire sauce and soup in slow cooker. Cover and cook over low heat for 6 to 8 hours. About 15 minutes before serving, add grated cheddar cheese and hot cooked pasta. Taste and add salt and pepper if necessary.

Serves 4 to 6.
Per serving: 479 calories; 2g fat; 48g protein; 67g carbohydrates; 6g dietary fibre; 51mg cholesterol; 809mg sodium.

Poulet Crockpot au fromage

2 lbs boneless skinless chicken breasts 2 cans
98% fat-free cream of chicken soup 1 can of
cheddar cheese soup
1/4 teaspoon garlic powder

Cut chicken into bite-sized pieces. Put the chicken in the bottom of the slow cooker. Add the rest of the ingredients to the top. Cook for 8 hours over low heat. Serve over rice or noodles.

Per serving: 328 calories; 8g fat; 55g protein; 5g carbohydrates; 1g dietary fibre; 146mg Cholesterol; 631mg sodium.

Chicken and Macaroni w/mushrooms

1 (10 3/4 oz) can Healthy Demand Cream of Chicken Soup 1/4 cup
Land O Lakes fat-free sour cream
16 oz uncooked and peeled chicken breast, cut into 20 pieces 1 cup (one 4 oz. can) sliced mushrooms, drained
1/2 cup finely chopped onion
1 1/3 cups (3 oz) uncooked elbow macaroni

Spray a slow cooker container with butter-flavoured cooking spray. In the prepared container, combine chicken soup and sour cream. Stir in chicken, mushrooms and onion. Add uncooked macaroni. Mix well to combine. Cover and cook on LOW for 6 to 8 hours. Stir gently again just before serving.

For 4 (1 cup) - Each serving à: equals: 263 Calories, 3 gm Fa, 26 gm Pr, Ca,542 mg So, 39 mg Cl,2 gm Fi

Chicken and rice

1/2 lb mushrooms, fresh
1/2 tse onion
1 lb chicken pieces
1 tsp chicken broth
1 tsp poultry seasoning 1/4
teaspoon salt
2 cs. water
3/4 ts rice, uncooked

Slice the mushrooms. Remove skin from chicken. Spray the 12-inch pan with non-stick coating. Brown mushrooms, onion and chicken pieces on all sides over medium heat for about 15 minutes. Stir in seasonings and transfer to slow cooker. Can be refrigerated overnight. Start the crockpot on LOW. When the ingredients are heated, add the rice. Cook until finished.

Makes 6 servings. Calories... 265...Fat... 6g... Protein... 25g... Carbohydrates... 27 g... Fiber... 0g.

Chicken A King Of La

1/4 cup onion -- finely chopped 1/4
cup celery -- finely chopped
1/4 cup green pepper -- finely chopped 1/4
cup chilli - chopped
4 ounces stems and pieces of mushrooms - drained
3 cups chicken or turkey -- cooked and cubed 1/2
teaspoon seasoned salt
1/8 teaspoon pepper
1 10 ounces mushroom soup   c cream
1 13 ounces evaporated skimmed milk

Put all ingredients in an electric slow cooker; mix. Cover and cook over low heat for 2 to 3 hours, or until well heated; stir once. Serve in patty shells or on warm fluffy rice. To reduce fat in this dish, use Campbell's Healthy Choice mushroom cream, fat-free cooked chicken breast meat, non-greasy evaporated milk and serve on white or brown rice cooked without adding.
Fat.   6 served

Chicken and stuffing

6 skinless skinless chicken breasts without skin
1 can of pan top stuffing mixture
1 can 98% fat-free cream of mushroom soup - or any cream soup 1/2 cup
water or chicken broth

Spray a 3 1/2 quarter crockpot with a cooking spray. Add chicken breasts. Combine stuffing, soup and liquid. Spread over chicken. Cook at low 6 - 8 hours.

Per serving: 321 calories; 6g fat; 56g protein; 7g carbohydrates; 1g dietary fibre; 137mg Cholesterol; 459mg sodium.

Brunswick Stew Chicken

2 tbsp flour
2 t instant broth granules, chicken flavor
1 1/2 teaspoons poultry
seasoning 1/4 teaspoon
pepper.
6 bones in chicken thighs (about 2 lbs))
Two med. potatoes cut into 1 1/2-
inch pieces of chopped onion
1 (15 oz) tomato sauce
1 T Worcestershire
1 (9 oz) pkg. haricots giant frozen baby beans lima, thawed 1 (9 oz)
pkg. frozen green giant corn niblets,, thawed

In a large resalableplasticbag, combine flour, broth, poultry seasoning and pepper; mix well. Add chicken thighs, potatoes and onion; seal bag and shake to coat. Place in slow cooker. In a small bowl, combine tomato sauce and Worcestershire sauce; mix well. Pour over chicken and vegetables in a slow cooker; stir gently to mix. Cover; cook over low heat for 7 hours. Stir in beans and corn. Cover up cook over low heat for another 30 minutes. To serve, remove bones from chicken thighs. Stir chicken into stew mixture; mix well. Makes 6 servings:
290 cal; 6g fat; 50 mg cholesterol; 550 mg sodium; 40g carbohydrates; 6g fibre; 20g protein.

Casablanca Chicken

2 tablespoons olive oil
2 large onions -- slice
1 teaspoon fresh ginger -- grater
3 Cl garlic -- chop
3 pounds boneless skinless chicken breasts
3 large carrots -- diced
2 large potatoes; peel -- dice
2 tablespoons Grapes 1/2
teaspoon Cumin 1/2
teaspoon turmeric
1/2 teaspoon Salt and pepper
1/4 teaspoon cinnamon
1/4 teaspoon cayenne pepper
1 can chopped tomatoes -- (14 1/2 ounces)
3 medium zucchini -- 1-inch slice
1 Can garbanzo beans -- (15 ounces) drain
2 tablespoons parsley -- chop 1/2
teaspoon Cilantro

Sauté onions, ginger and garlic in oil. Transfer to the crockpot. Brown chicken in the same skillet over medium heat. Add carrots, potatoes and zucchini to slow cooker. Place chicken on top of vegetables. Stir seasonings into a small brown and sprinkle with chicken. Add raisins and tomatoes. Cover and cook on HIGH for 4 to 6 hours. Add beans, parsley and coriander 30 minutes before serving. Serve over cooked rice or couscous.
Source: Rival.

Per serving: 380 calories; 7g fat; 47g protein; 31g carbohydrates; 7g dietary fibre; 99mg Cholesterol; 223mg sodium.

Chicken Cordon Bleu

4-6 chicken breasts (battered)
4-6 pieces ham
4-6 slices Swiss cheese or mozzarella
1 can of mushroom soup cream (can use any cream soup) 1/4 cup
milk

Place ham and cheese on chicken. Roll and fix with a toothpick. Place the chicken in the slow cooker so that it looks like a triangle/ Layer the rest on top. Mix soup with milk; pour over the top of the chicken. Cover and cook over low heat for 4 hours or until chicken is no longer pink. Serve over noodles with the sauce it makes.
Note: This is the best recipe I've tried so far, very tasty.

Chicken dinner in a Crock-Pot

4 boneless skinless chicken breasts
2 tsp dried basil
1/8 teaspoon salt and
pepper 1 cup diced pepper
1 (16 oz) can white beans, drained and rinsed
1 (14 oz) canned tomatoes, not

Put the chicken in a slow cookery jar: sprinkle with basil and salt and pepper. Add pepper, beans and tomatoes. Cover with lid; cook at low setting for 8 hours. The serving is 1 chicken breast with 1 cup of tomato bean mixture. PORTIONS: 4

Chicken in mushroom sauce

6 boneless whole skinless chicken breasts
21 1/2 ounces 98% fat-free condensed cream of mushroom soup to taste
Salt and pepper
8 Oz mushrooms, canned - sliced and drained 1/2
cup dry white wine

Place chicken breasts in slow cooker. Season with salt and pepper. Combine wine and soup. Pour over chicken. Add mushrooms. Cover. Cook on LOW for 7 to 9 hours.

Chicken Italiano

1 pound boneless, skinless chicken thighs
1 medium onion -- chopped
1/2 cup pitted ripe olives -- halved 2
tablespoons capers
1 teaspoon dried oregano leaves 1/2
teaspoon salt
1/2 teaspoon dried rosemary leaves -- crushed 1/4
teaspoon garlic powder
2 cups diced canned tomatoes -- un arrowed 1/4
cup water
1 tablespoon cornstarch

Place chicken in a slow cooker of 3-1/2 to 4 quarters. Garnish with onion, olives and capers. Sprinkle with oregano, salt, rosemary and garlic powder. Pour tomatoes over chicken. Cover; cook at low setting for 7 to 10 hours or until chicken is tender with a fork, juice is clear and onion is tender. Remove chicken and vegetables from slow cooker with a slotted spoon; place on the serving tray. Cover to warm up. In a small bowl, combine water and cornstarch; mix well. Add to slow cooker. Increase the setting to a high level; cook until thickened. Serve with chicken.

4 Portions.
Per serving: 246 calories; 12g fat; 74g protein; 11g carbohydrates; 2g dietary fibre; 57mg cholesterol; 705mg sodium.

Service Ideas: This chicken is delicious served on pasta.

Chicken noodle soup

3/4 pound boneless, skinless chicken thighs -- cut into 1-inch pieces 2
cups sliced celery -- (2 medium stems)
2 cups chopped carrots
3/4 cup chopped onion -- (1 medium)
14 1/2 ounces ready-to-serve chicken broth -- (1 can) 1/2
teaspoon dried marjoram -- crushed
1 teaspoon dried thyme leaves - crushed 1/2
teaspoon salt - optional
2 bay leaves
10 ounces frozen green peas -- (1 pkg.)
1 cup homemade frozen egg noodles

Spray the 10-inch skillet with cooking spray; heat over medium heat. Cook chicken in skillet for 5 minutes, stirring frequently, until golden brown. Mix chicken and remaining ingredients, except peas and noodles in a slow 3 1/2 to 4 litre stove. Cover and cook over low heat for 6 and a half to 7 hours or until chicken is no longer pink in the centre. Stir in peas and noodles; cook for about 10 minutes more or until noodles are tender.

Per serving: 218 calories; 6g fat; 42g protein; 24g Carbohydrates; 5g dietary fibre; 41mg Cholesterol; 601mg sodium.

Chicken noodle soup#2

1 whole chicken, no skin, cut
2 medium carrots -- peeled and chopped 1/2 cup onion -- peeled and chopped
2 Stalks celery - coarsely chopped
2 1/2 teaspoons salt
2 teaspoons parsley 3/4 teaspoon marjoram 1/2 teaspoon basil
1/4 teaspoon poultry seasoning 1/4 teaspoon pepper
1 Bay leaf
2 qt Water
2 1/2 cups egg noodles

Place the first 4 ingredients in a 3 1/2-quarter slow cooker quart in the order indicated. Mix salt and the following 6 ingredients; sprinkle over vegetables. Add 6 cups of water; cover and cook at low setting for 8 to 10 hours. Remove chicken and bay leaf; add the remaining 2 cups of water. Stir in noodles and cook, covered, over high heat for 20 minutes. Meanwhile, remove the bones from the chicken and cut the chicken into bite-sized pieces. Add to slow cooker, stir to mix. Bake for 15 minutes, covered or until noodles are tender. Makes 3 quarters 1/4. Serves 8 to 10.

Per serving: 63 Calories; 1g fat (10% calories from fat); 3g protein; 12g carbohydrates; 13mg cholesterol; 693mg sodium

Chicken paella

1 LB(s) boneless Tyson, skinless chicken thighs, or similar product (four 4 ozthighs) 2 medium tomatoes, chopped
1 medium onion, chopped
1 medium green pepper, chopped 1/2 cup chicken stock
3 medium garlic cloves, chopped
1 tsp dried oregano
1 tsp ground turmeric
1/3 cup (s) frozen green peas 2 cups (s) cooked white rice

Place chicken, tomatoes, onion, pepper, broth, garlic, oregano and turmeric in a slow cookery of 4-quarters or more (crockpot). Cover and cook at low setting for 5 hours. Add peas and rice; cook, uncovered, until peas are tender, about 15 minutes. Makes about 1 1/2 cups per serving (including 1 chicken leg per serving).

Servit, 4

Chicken Parmesan
Donne 4 portions Med. Crockery Pot

2 tsp olive oil

4 skinless, boneless chicken breasts (about 3 oz) each

1 1/4 cups crushed tomatoes
2 large garlic cloves, crushed
1 tsp sugar
Pinch celery seeds 2 tbsp
dry red wine
1/2 cup grated mozzarella cheese 2 tbsp
grated Parmesan cheese

Heat oil in a non-stick skillet over low heat. Add chicken and sauté, stirring occasionally, until lightly browned, about 10 min. Mix chicken and next 5 ingredients in pot. Cover and cook on LOW until chicken is cooked through and meat thermometer is 170th; 6-8 hours. Mix the cheeses in a small bowl and sprinkle over the chicken. Don't move. Cook until cheeses are melted, about 15 minutes.

Per serving: 249cal, 8.3g fat, 364mg turf, 1.3g fib

Chicken stew

1 pound of boneless and peeled chicken breasts
1 pound of boneless and peeled chicken thighs
2 cups water
1 cup frozen whole onions
1 cup sliced celery -- (1/2 inch)
1 cup finely sliced carrots
1 teaspoon paprika
1/2 teaspoon salt
1/2 teaspoon rubbed sage 1/2
teaspoon dried thyme 1/2
teaspoon pepper
1 (10 ounces) can Ro tomatoesand chillies-Tel
1 (14 1/4 ounces) can fat-free chicken broth
2 cups of mushrooms cut in half
1 (6 ounces) can stick tomato 1/4
cup water
3 tablespoons cornstarch
2 cups frozen green peas

Mix the first 15 ingredients in a large electric slow cooker. Cover with lid and cook over high heat for 4 hours or until carrot is tender. Mix the water and cornstarch in a small bowl, stirring with a metal whisk until mixed. Add cornstarch mixture and peas to slow cooker; stir well. Cover and cook over high heat, 30 minutes more.

(servingsize: 1-1/2 cups)
Per serving (excluding unknown items): 178 calories; 3g fat (16.5% calories from fat); 22g protein; 17g carbohydrates; 4g dietary fibre; 48mg Cholesterol; 512mg sodium.

Poulet Stroganoff

1 pound boneless, skinless frozen chicken breasts
1 can of fat-free cream of mushroom soup
16 oz fat-free sour cream cardboard
1 slice of dry onion soup mixture

Place frozen chicken in bottom of slow cooker. Mix the soup, sour cream, onion soup mixture and pour over the chicken, Cook over low heat for 7 hours. Makes 6 servings. (Serveservez-le it on rice or noodles)

6 Portions

Poulet Stroganoff #2

1 cup fat-free sour cream
1 tablespoon all-purpose gold metal flour
1 slice of chicken sauce mixture - (.87 to 1.2 oz.) 1
cup water
1 pound skinless boneless chicken breast -- cut into 1-inch 16-ounce
frozen california frozen vegetable pieces -- thawed
1 cup sliced and sautéed mushrooms
1 cup frozen peas
10 ounces potatoes -- peeled to 1" pieces (about 2 potatoes, weight after peeled) 1 1/2 cups Bisquick® cooking mixture
4 green onions -- chopped (1/3 cup) 1/2
cup low-fat milk

Combine sour cream, flour, sauce mixture and water in a slow cookery Crock-Pot from 3-1/2 to 4 quarters until smooth. Stir in chicken, vegetables and mushrooms. Cover and cook over low heat for 4 hours or until tender chicken and sauce are thickened. Stir in peas. Mix the pastry mixture and onions. Stir in milk until moistened. Place dough with des rounded tablespoons on chicken-vegetable mixtures. Cover and cook over high heat for 45 to 50 minutes or until toothpick inserted in centre of meatballs is clean. Serve 4 servings immediately.

NOTES: Save time To cut chicken into pieces and chop green onions the day before. Pack them separately and store them in the refrigerator.

Poulet Stroganoff Suprême

1 cup fat-free sour cream
1 tablespoon all-purpose flour
1 chicken wrap with mixed sauce
1 cup water
1 boneless skinless chicken breast halves - cut into 1" 16-ounce pieces of
frozen stew vegetables - thawed
4 ounces pieces of mushrooms - drained
1 cup frozen green peas -- thawed
1 1/2 cups bisquick.cooking mixture
4 whole green onions 1/2
cup skimmed milk

Combine sour cream, all-purpose flour, sauce mixture and water in a slow cookery for 3 1/2 to 4 quarters until smooth. Stir in chicken, stewed vegetables and mushrooms. Cover and cook over low heat for 5 hours or until chicken is tender and sauce thickens. Stir in peas. Mix the cooking mixture and the green onions. Stir in milk until moistened. Place the dough with rounded tablespoons on the chicken-vegetable mixture. Cover and cook over high heat for 45-50 minutes or until toothpick inserted in centre of meatballs comes out clean. Serve immediately.

Per serving: 406 calories; 8g fat; 37g protein; 46g carbohydrates; 4g dietary fibre; 73mg Cholesterol; 786mg sodium.

Vegetarian chicken soup

1 1/2 boneless, skinless chicken breast
3 carrots, diced
3 potatoes - diced
1 onion, chopped
2 cups anise root - chopped
2 cups cabbage -- chopped
10 ounces low-fat chicken broth -- 1 can Campbell's
5 cans of water - just enough to cover
2 bay leaves
Salt and pepper - to taste of
garlic - to taste
Italian seasoning - to taste
3 chillies - dried removed when - made

Cook over low heat for about 8-10 hours (until vegetables are cooked) Per serving: 82.9 cal, 0.7g (6.9%) fat, 1.5g fibre, 113 mg sodium

Chicken-vegetable chowds

Service size: 5

1 pound boneless skinless chicken thighs -- cut into 1" 1 cup fresh
carrots, halved -- lengthwise
1 cup sliced fresh mushrooms 1/2
cup chopped onion
1/2 cup water
1/4 teaspoon garlic powder
1/8 teaspoon dried thyme leaves
1 14 1/2 oz ready-to-serve chicken broth
1 10 3/4oz.can condensed cream of chicken and broccoli soup -- 98% fat-free, with 30% less sodium

1/2 cup milk
3 tablespoons all-purpose flour

1 9 oz pkg. Green Giant Harvest Fresh Cut Broccoli -- thawed

In a 3 1/2 to 4-quarter Crock-Pot slow cooker, combine chicken, carrots, mushrooms, onion, water, garlic powder, thyme and broth; mix well. Cover; cook at low setting for 7 to 9 hours or until chicken is no longer pink. Drain the fat from the slow cooker. In a small bowl, combine soup, milk and flour; beat with metal whisk until smooth. Add soup mixture and broccoli to chicken mixture. Cover; cook for another 30 minutes or until broccoli is tender.

5 servings of 1 1/2 cups. Per serving: 220 Cal; Total fat 5g; (Satsam 2g); Choles 60mg; Sod 660mg; Total carbohydrates 17g; 3g fiber; Sugars 5g; Pro 26g.

Chicken wings in BBQ sauce

3 pounds chicken wings - about 16 wings Salt
and pepper - to taste
1 1/2 cups barbecue sauce -- any variety 1/4
cup honey
2 teaspoons prepared mustard - or spicy mustard
2 teaspoons Worcestershire sauce Hot
pepper sauce - to taste, optional

Rinse chicken and dry. Cut and discard the ends of the wing. Cut each wing to the joint to make two sections. Place the wing parts on the grilling pan. Grill 4 to 5 inches roma heat for 20 minutes, 10 minutes sided or until chicken is brown. Transfer chicken to Crock-Pot Slow Cooker. For the sauce, combine barbecue sauce, honey, mustard, Worcestershire sauce and hot pepper sauce, if desired, in a small bow. Pour over chicken wings. Cover and cook on low for 4 to 5 hours or 2 to 2 and a half hours. Serve directly from Crock-Pot Slow Cooker.
Per serving: 61 Calories; 3g total fat; 4g protein; 3g carbohydrates; 16mg cholesterol; 106mg sodium

Chicken wings in honey sauce

3 pounds chicken wings - about 16 wings Salt
and pepper - to taste
2 cups honey
1 cup low-sodium soy sauce 1/2
cup ketchup
1/4 cup oil
Sesame seeds -- optional

Rinse chicken and dry. Cut and discard the ends of the wing. Cut each wing to the joint to make two sections. Place the wing parts on the grilling pan. Grill 4 to 5 inches of heat for 20 minutes, 10 minutes side-on or until chicken is brown. Transfer chicken to Crock-Pot Slow Cooker. For the sauce, combine honey, soy sauce, ketchup, oil and garlic in a bowl. Pour over chicken wings. Cover and cook on low for 4 to 5 hours or 2 to 2 and a half hours. Garnish with sesame seeds, if desired.
Per serving: 124 calories; 5g total fat; 4g protein; 17g carbohydrates; 16mg cholesterol; 322mg sodium

Chicken wings with Teriyaki sauce

3-pound chicken wings - about 16 wings
1 large onion, chopped
1 cup brown sugar
1 cup low-sodium soy sauce
1/4 cup dry sherry -- or chicken broth 2
teaspoons ground ginger
2 garlic cloves, chopped

Rinse chicken and dry. Cut and discard the ends of the wing. Cut each wing to the joint to make two sections. Place the wing parts on the grilling pan. Grill 4 to 5 inches of heat for 20 minutes, 10 minutes side-on or until chicken is brown. Transfer chicken to Crock-Pot Slow Cooker. Combine onion, brown sugar, soy sauce, sherry (or chicken broth), ginger and garlic in a bowl. Pour over chicken wings. Cover and cook at low 5 to 6 hours or on High 2 to 3 hours. Stir the chicken wings once to make sure the wings are evenly coated with sauce. Serve from Crock-Pot Slow Cooker.
Per serving: 68 Calories); (kcal); 3g total fat; 4g protein; 5g carbohydrates; 16mg Chol;283mg sodium 7l

Chicken with Lima beans C/P

1 fried whole chicken -- cut to taste
Salt
To taste Pepper 1
tablespoon oil
2 large potatoes -- cubed
1 package frozen Lima beans -- thawed
1 cup chicken broth 1/4
teaspoon thyme

Season chicken with salt and pepper. Heat oil and butter in a large frying pan. Fry chicken on both sides until golden. Add to slow cooker with remaining ingredients. Cover and cook over low heat for 4 to 6 hours.

Chile

1 Livre Ground Sirloin
2 cans red beans
1 large tomato juice can, low sodium -- V8
1 small-headed cabbage -- sliced
1 medium onion -- chopped
1 small tomato can -- chopped, optional
1 Pinch salt -- optional
1 teaspoon chili powder -- (1 to 2)

This can be cooked on the stove or in a slow cooker. Put the V-8 juice in the pan or slow cooker. Now brown the ground beef and add to the juice. You can now add the rest of the ingredients. Cook until cabbage is cooked or to consistency, you wish. Stir from time to time. You can serve this on rice and you can also sprinkle with cheese. It's really good.

Chili Mac Pot

16 ounces ground turkey or extra lean beef
1 cup chopped onion
2 cups (a 16-ounce can) tomatoes, coarsely chopped and not
1 (10 3/4 ounces) can demand healthy tomato soup
1 cup reduced sodium tomato juice
2 teaspoons chili seasoning
6 ounces (an 8-ounce can) of red beans, rinsed and drained
1 cup macaroni at the elbow

In a large frying pan sprayed with olive oil flavored cooking spray, brown meat. Meanwhile, in a slow cooker container sprayed with cooking spray, combine onion, non-dramatic tomatoes, tomato soup, tomato juice and chili seasoning. Stir in red beans and uncooked macaroni. Add the browned meat. Mix well to combine. Cover and cook on LOW for 6 to 8 hours. Mix well before serving.

Serves 6 (1 full cup)

Chili Pasta Cook

Makes 7 servings (1 cup)

1 1/2 lbs lean ground beef
1 cup chopped onion
2 (14 oz) cans of tomatoes with juice, crushed
2 tsp chili powder
1/2 tsp dried whole oregano 7.5
oz tomato juice
1 tsp salt
1/4 teaspoon pepper
1 1/4 cups uncooked elbow macaroni
1 cup Monterey Jack cheese (or med. Cheddar) grated

Mix ground beef in a non-stick skillet until golden. Drain well. Transfer to 3 1/2 qt. slow cooker. Add the nest 8 ingredients. Stir. Cover. Cook over low heat for 5-7 hours. or on HIGH for 2 1/2-3 1/2 hours. Sprinkle cheese on top. Cook on HIGH for 10 to 15 minutes until cheese is melted.

Per serving: 329cal, 14g fat, 904 mg turf, 28g prot,25g carbohydrates

Chinese beef and pea pods

1 pound flank steak
10 1/2 ounces beef consumed 1/4
cup soy sauce
1/4 teaspoon ground ginger
1 bunch green onions - sliced
2 tablespoons cornstarch
2 tablespoons cold water
7 ounces snow peas - frozen, partially thawed

Finely slice the steak from the side diagonally over the grain. Mix the strips in a slow-cooked saucepan with consummate, soy sauce, ginger and onions. Cover and cook over low heat for 5 to 7 hours. Turn the control to the height. Stir in cornstarch that has been dissolved in cold water. Cook over high heat for 10 to 15 minutes or until thickened. Place in pea pods for the last 5 minutes. Service Ideas: Serve on hot rice.

Chinese beef and vegetable stew

6 portions

4 cups shredded cabbage, packaged
1 large green pepper -- cut into thin strips 4 1/2
ounces canned mushrooms -- 1 jar
6 shallots - chopped
1 can, (8 ounces) water chestnut, canned - drained
1 pound lean round steak - cut into strips 1/4
cup dry sherry
3 tablespoons soy sauce
3 tablespoons water
3 tablespoons hoisin sauce
1 teaspoon Chinese chili paste with garlic 1/4
teaspoon garlic powder
1/4 teaspoon pepper
1 1/2 tablespoons cornstarch
16 ounces frozen young green beans, thawed 1/2
large red pepper, chopped

In a 3 1/2- or 4-quarter electric slow cooker, combine cabbage, green pepper, mushrooms, green onions, water chestnuts and beef. In a small bowl, combine 2 tablespoons each of sherry and soy sauce, water hoisine sauce, chili paste and garlic powder. Pour over beef and vegetables in saucepan. Sprinkle with garlic pepper. Cover and cook over low heat for 5 and a half to 6 hours. In a small bowl or cup, combine cornstarch and remaining sherry and soy sauce. Increase the heat setting to high. Stir in cornstarch mixture. Place lid slightly ajar and cook over high heat for 1/2 hour, stirring once or twice, until sauce clears and thickens slightly. Stir in green beans and red pepper and cook for another 5 to 10 minutes.

Per serving (excluding unknown items): 197 Calories; 4g fat (20.3% calories from fat); 20g protein; 18g carbohydrates; 5g dietary fibre; 44mg Cholesterol; 794mg sodium.

NOTES: Chinese aromas and a blend of Asian and regular vegetables give this stew a contemporary east-west touch. Serve over steamed hot rice. Use a 4-quarter slow cooker and stir in 1 to 2 cups of bean sprouts with the cabbage, if desired.

Chops in a jar of Crock

6 whole pork loin chops -- browned
1 whole onion - chopped
3 Catsup TB
10 1/2 oz 98%fat-free Chicken soup cream 2 Ts
Worcestershire sauce

Put everything in a slow cooker and cook on LOW for about 4-5 hours. Serve with rice, noodles or potatoes.

For 6 servings: 154 calories; 6g fat; 21g protein; 8g carbohydrates; 1g dietary fibre; 51mg cholesterol; 479mg sodium.

Chop Suey on Rice
Makes 5 servings

1 lb boneless pork shoulder, cut into 3/4' cubes
1 small onion, cut into 1/4-inch wedges
1 (5oz) can slices of bamboo shoots, drained 1/2
cup purchased teriyaki baste and glaze 1 tsp
grated ginger
1 (1 lb) pkg. frozen broccoli, carrots and water chestnuts, thawed, drained 2 cups
raw instant white rice
2 cups water

In 4-6 qt. slow cooker, mix the first 6 ingredients; mix well. Cover; cook on LOW for 5-7 hours. About 15 minutes before serving, add the vegetables to the pork. Increase heat setting to high; cover and cook for 10-15 minutes more or until vegetables are tender. Meanwhile, cook the rice in water as shown on pkg. Serve pork mixture over rice.

Per serving: Cal 430, fat 14 g, sat fat 5 g, chol 55 mg, turf 1180 mg, carbohydrates 54 g, fib 3 g, prot 21 g

Chunky Boeuf et Chili de porc

1 pound beef round steak
1 pound pork shoulder steak
1 large onion -- chopped (1 cup)
2 garlic cloves -- finely chopped
15 ounces stocky tomato sauce
12 ounces thick, thick salsa
2 teaspoons Mexican seasoning
1 medium green pepper -- chopped (1 cup) sour
cream -- (optional)
Cheddar cheese -- grated (optional)

Remove excess fat from beef and pork. Cut beef and pork into 3/4-inch pieces. Combine beef, pork and remaining ingredients, except pepper, sour cream and cheese in a slow 3 1/2 to 6 litre stove. Cover and cook over low heat for 8 to 10 hours or until pork is tender. Stir in pepper. Cover and cook over low heat for 15 to 30 minutes or until pepper is tender. Serve chili topped with sour cream and cheese if desired.

Per serving: cals 215;fat 8 g; chol 70 mg; sodium 620 mg; carbohydrates 12 g; fiber 3 g; protein 27 g

Cola-chicken

1 cup Cola -- regular
1 cup Catsup
1 whole onion - sliced
1 1/2 pounds boneless skinless chicken breast

Wash and pat the dry chicken. Season with salt and pepper to taste. Put the chicken in the slow cooker and the onions on top. Add cola and catsup and cook on LOW for 6 to 8 hours. Once cooked place in the refrigerator to cool, then skim the fat. Warm up and eat. Sounds horrible --- but believe me on what taste ---- isWONDERFUL!!!!

Per serving: 286 calories; 2g fat; 41g protein; 25g carbohydrates; 1g dietary fibre; 99mg Cholesterol; 826mg sodium.

Colorful chicken stew

1 lb   boneless skinless chicken breasts, cubed
1 can 14 1/2 oz   Italian diced tomatoes, not
2 medium potatoes, peeled and cut into half-inch cubes 5
medium carrots, chopped
3 celery ribs, chopped
1 large onion, chopped
1 medium green pepper, chopped
2 cans (4 oz each) of mushroom stems and pieces, drained
2 cubes low-sodium chicken broth
2 tsp sugar (I used Splenda))
1 tsp chili powder 1/4
teaspoon pepper
1 tbsp cornstarch
2 cups cold water

In a 5 qt slow cooker, combine the first 12 ingredients. In a small bowl, combine cornstarch and water until smooth. Stir in chicken mixture. Cover and cook over low heat for 8 to 10 hours or until vegetables are tender.

Yield 10 servings 1 cup serving 123 calories,209 mg sodium, 25 mg cholesterol, 16 gmcarbohydrates, 11 grmproteins,, 1 gm fat, , 3 gm   fibers. .

Crock Pot Chili comforting

1 pound ground turkey breast or very lean ground beef 1 large
onion - finely chopped
5 oz   pinto beans -- rinsed and drained
8 1/2 oz   corn -- rinsed and drained
15 oz   tomato sauce
14 1/2 oz   diced tomatoes
10 oz   diced tomatoes and green peppers
1 tbsp chili powder
1 tsp ground cumin 1/2
teaspoon garlic powder
1/2 teaspoon salt.

In a non-stick skillet over medium heat, cook ground meat until meat is no longer pink; Aspire. Transfer the meat to Crock Pot. Add remaining ingredients and stir until smooth. Cook on "high" for 4 hours; remove the lid and stir quickly halfway.

Yield 8 cups Serving size: 1 cup per serving: Calories: 214, Carbohydrates: 24g, Protein: 16g, Fat: 6g, Saturated Fat: 2g, Sodium: 901 mg, Fibre: 5g

Rooster with wine

4 slices of bacon, cut thick
2 cups frozen pearl onions -- thawed
1 cup mushrooms button - sliced
1 clove garlic - chopped
1 teaspoon dried thyme leaves 1/8
teaspoon black pepper
2 pounds boneless skinless chicken breast halves - 6 - 5 oz.pieces 1 cup dry
red wine
3/4 cup reduced sodium chicken broth 1/4
cup tomato paste
3 tablespoons all-purpose flour

Cook bacon in a medium skillet over medium heat. Drain and collapse. Spread the ingredients in the slow cooker in the following order. onions,bacon, mushrooms, garlic, thyme, pepper, chicken, wine and broth. Cover and cook on LOW 6 to 8 hours. Remove chicken and vegetables; cover and keep warm. Roll the cooking liquid into a small bowl; allow to cool slightly. Turn the slow cooker into a HIGH; Cover. Mix the reserved liquid, tomato paste and flour until smooth. Return the mixture to the slow cooker; cover and cook for 15 minutes or until thickened. Serve over egg noodles, if desired.

Makes 6 servings
Per serving: 293 calories; 6g fat; 40g protein; 11g carbohydrates; 2g dietary fibre; 95mg Cholesterol; 446mg sodium.

Scallops of corn, ham and potato

6 cups peeled cooked potatoes -- cut into 1.1/2-inch
cubes of cubed ham
1 15.25oz. Green Giant Whole Kernel Sweet Corn - drained 1/4 cup
chopped green pepper
2 teaspoons instant chopped onion
1 10 3/4oz.can condensed cheddar cheese sauce 1/2
cup milk
2 tablespoons all-purpose flour

In a 3 1/2 to 4-quarter Crock-Pot slow cooker, combine potatoes, ham, corn, pepper and onion; mix well. In a small bowl, combine soup, milk and flour; beat with metal whisk until smooth. Pour soup mixture over potato mixture; terre; stir gently to mix. Cover; cook at low setting for 7 to 9 hours or until potatoes are tender.

Info: Potatoes cook faster when cut into small pieces; cubed potatoes will cook faster than quartered potatoes. The 1 inch potato pieces in our recipe work well as they don't get too soft during the long cooking period. In addition, leftover cooked beef or turkey roast can be used in place of ham.

6 servings of 6 servings and 1 1/2 cups. Per serving: Cal 320; Total fat 7g; (Satsam 4g); Choles 30mg; Sod 1010mg; Total carbohydrates 49g; 5g fibre; Sugars 6g; Pro 14g.

Horned beef hash

3 cups corned beef breast - cooked
2 small onions, chopped
3 potatoes, chopped
1 teaspoon salt
1/2 teaspoon pepper
1 cup low-fat beef stock

Run the first three ingredients through the food grinder (food robot?). Mix well with all the remaining ingredients. Squeeze into greased jar. Cover and cook on LOW for 8 to 10 hours.
Per serving: 297 Calories); (kcal); 18g total fat; (52% calories from fat); 21g protein; 15g carbohydrates; 63mg Cholesterol; 589 mg sodium

Country captain chicken with rice
Number of servings: 4

2 cups sliced shiitake mushrooms
1 cup chopped onion 1/2
cup chopped celery 1
clove garlic, finely
chopped
1 LB (450g) boneless, skinless chicken thighs, cut from all fats and cut into bite-sized pieces 1 tbsp flour.
1/4 cup fat-free chicken broth 1
1/2 teaspoons curry powder
1 tsp salt
1/4 teaspoon
pepper 1/4
teaspoon. Paprika
3 cups canned crushed tomatoes 1/4
cup golden raisins
2 cups cooked brown rice

Coat a large frying pan with cooking spray. Add mushrooms, onion, celery and garlic and sauté until vegetables are tender, about 5 minutes. Put the vegetables in a slow cooker; add the chicken. In a cup, mix flour and chicken broth until smooth. Add to slow cooker. Add curry powder, salt, pepper, paprika, crushed tomatoes and raisins, and stir in. Cover and cook over low heat for 5 hours. To serve, pour 1/2 cup of rice on each of the 4 plates. Garnish each with chicken and sauce and serve. Makes 2 1/2 cups of chicken mixture and 1/2 cup of rice per serving.

Nutritional Profile per Serving: Calories 377.8, Protein 30.7g, Fat 6.6g, Saturated Fat 1.5g, Carbohydrates 50.3g, Fibre 7.2g, Cholesterol 94.1mg, Iron 4.8mg, Sodium 1044.4mg, Calcium 108.3mg

Cowboy stew
Makes 6 servings

1 1/4 lbs beef stew
4 potatoes, unpeeled, cut into 4-inch pcs
1/2 cup onion, chopped
1 tsp salt
1/4 teaspoon pepper
1 (28 oz) baked beans in BBQ sauce

Combine beef, potatoes, onion, salt and pepper in 3 1/2 qt. à 4 qt. slow cooker. Spread beans over beef mixture. Cover and cook on LOW 8-10 hours. or until the beef is tender.

Per serving: cal 370, fat 12g, fat sat 5g, chol 65mg, turf 1030mg, carbohydrates 46g, fiber 8g, prot 28g

Confortable Crock Comfort Serves-6

16 oz ground 90% lean turkey or beef 1/2
cup chopped onion
3 cups (15oz) raw potatoes, diced 1/3
cup (1 oz) raw regular rice 1 1/2 cups
grated carrots
1 cup celery, finely diced
1 1/2 cups healthy-to-eat tomato juice or any reduced-sodium tomato juice 1 (10 3/4 oz)
may require healthy-in-demand tomato soup
1/4 teaspoon black pepper
1 tsp dried parsley flakes

In a large frying pan sprayed with butter-flavoured spray, brown meat. Place the browned meat in a slow cooker container. Add onion, potatoes, uncooked rice, carrots and celery. Mix well to combine. Stir in tomato juice, tomato soup, black pepper and parsley flakes. Cover and cook on LOW for 6 to 8 hours. Mix well before serving.

Each serving is equal: 243 Calories, 7gm Fat, 16gm Pro., 29gm Carbo, 290mg Sodium, 33mg Calcium, 3gm Fiber

Creamy chicken and wild rice

1 pkg. (8.25 oz) mushroom and wild rice pan-dinner mix 1 lb, skinless
and boneless chicken breast, cut into 1 pcs.
1 can (14 1/2 oz) ready-to-serve chicken broth 1 can
(12 oz) evaporated milk
1/2 cup water
2 tbsp margarine or butter, melted
2 tbsp instantly chopped onion

Mix the uncooked rice and sauce mixture (from the dinner mixture) and the rest of the ingredients in 2-3 1/2 qt. slow cooker. Cover and cook on LOW for 5 to 6 hours or until rice is tender. Stir the mixture. Cover and let stand for about 15 minutes or until thickened and desired consistency.

Per serving: cal 330, fat 11g, fat sat 3g, chol 80mg, turf 1250mg, carbohydrates 328mg, fiber 2g

Creamy red potatoes

2 Pounds of red potatoes - in quarters
8 Ounces Cheese Neufchatel
10 3/4 Ounces Potato Soup Cream
1 Wrap Ranch-style Dressing Mix

Put the potatoes in a slow cooker. Beat together the cream cheese, soup and dressing mixture. Stir in potatoes. Cover and cook over low heat for 8 hours or until potatoes are tender.

Per serving (excluding unknown items): 234 calories; 9g fat (35.9% calories from fat); 7g protein; 31g carbohydrates; 3g dietary fibre; 30mg cholesterol; 390mg sodium. Exchanges: 2 Grain (Starch); 1/2 Lean meat; 1 1/2 fat.

Creamy red potatoes and chicken

1 1/2 pounds of red potatoes -- in pieces
8 Ounces Cheese Neufchatel
10 3/4 Ounces Potato Soup Cream
1 Wrap Ranch-style Dressing Mix
12 Ounces skinless chicken breast - cut into strips

Put the potatoes in a slow cooker. Beat together the cream cheese, soup and dressing mixture. Stir in chicken strips and spread over potatoes (or simply stir together). Cover and cook over low heat for 8 hours or until potatoes are tender. Stir once after 5-6 hours. Stir before serving.

Per serving (excluding unknown items): 381 calories; 15g fat (35.5% calories from fat); 25g protein; 36g carbohydrates; 3g dietary fibre; 84mg Cholesterol; 626mg sodium.

Cooked pineapple chicken

6 whole halves of skinless chicken breast -- peeled and split 1
dashboard pepper
To taste the paprika
20 ounces pineapple pieces in juice - 1 treats 2
tablespoons Dijon mustard
2 tablespoons soy sauce
1 clove garlic - chopped

Arrange chicken at bottom of slow cooker. Sprinkle with pepper and paprika. In a small bowl, combine drained pineapple treats, mustard and soy sauce. Pour over chicken. Add chopped garlic. Cover and cook on LOW 7-9 hours or HIGH 3-4 hours. Makes 6 servings.

Per serving: 194 calories; 2g fat; 28g protein; 16g carbohydrates; 1g dietary fibre; 68mg Cholesterol; 483mg sodium.

Tarte aux pommes Crockpot

8 apples -- pie, peeled and sliced
1 1/4 teaspoon cinnamon 1/4
teaspoon chilli
1/4 teaspoon nutmeg
3/4 cup skimmed milk
2 tablespoons Brummel and Brown Spread - softened 3/4 cup
Splenda
1/2 cup egg mixers® 99% egg substitute 1
teaspoon vanilla extract
1/2 cup reduced Bisquickfat ® 1/3
cup brown sugar
3 tablespoons cold butter

Mix apples in a large bowl with cinnamon, chilli and nutmeg. Place in a lightly greased slow cooker. Combine milk, softened butter, sugar, eggs, vanilla and Bisquick 1/2de t. Pour over apples. Mix 1 cup Bisquick and brown sugar. Cut the cold butter into a mixture until it is crumbly. Sprinkle this mixture over the apple mixture. Cover and cook over low heat for 6 to 7 hours or until apples are tender.

Per serving: 200 calories; 7g fat; 4g dietary fibre

Crockpot Baked Beans

Service size: 10

1/2 medium onion -- chopped
5 slices of turkey bacon - chopped
4 ounces ground beef (80% lean)
1 can of vegetarian beans in tomato sauce - (16 oz) 1 can of beans with vegetarian bacon - (16 oz)
1 can of red beans - (16oz)-- rinsed, drained 1/2 cup tomato sauce
2 tablespoons brown sugar
1 teaspoon liquid smoke - (2 teaspoons)
1/2 teaspoon maple flavour

Lightly spray an unheated medium skillet with a stickless spray. Add onions and bacon. Cook and stir over medium-high heat until onions are tender. Add ground beef and cook until golden, stirring occasionally. Transfer the onion mixture to a slow cooker for 4 to 6 quarters. Stir beans with tomato sauce, baked beans, red beans, tomato sauce, brown sugar, liquid smoke and maple flavour. Cover and cook over medium-high heat for 4 to 6 hours (if necessary, adjust the heat setting so that the beans simmer slowly during cooking). Stir before serving.

Comments: Here is a hearty side dish that is always a favorite at picnics.
Nutritional information per serving: Calories: 206; Fat: 3 grams (14% of calories); Cholesterol: 15 milligrams; Sodium: 480 milligrams; Fibre (grams) 5.2.

Crockpot beef and peppers

Serves 8

2 lbs lean round steak, cut all fat
2 green peppers, thinly sliced
2 tbsp dried onions, 1 large used fresh onions 1 cup beef stock
2 tbsp low-sodium soy sauce
1 tsp Worcestershire sauce
1/2 tsp ground ginger (optional)
1 clove garlic, chopped (I used 4 cloves)

Cut steak into serving size pieces. Put the vegetables in the bottom of the slow cooker, then put the steak in a single layer on the vegetables. Pour the rest of the ingredients over the top. Cover and cook over low heat for 8 to 10 hours or high for about 4 hours. I found that I needed to add more water because it was so salty. Then when it was almost done, I thickened it with a little flour.

Boeuf et bouillon Crockpot

2 tablespoons vegetable oil
2 pounds beef shank crossed cuts or soup bones 5
cups cold water
1 1/4 teaspoons salt
1/4 teaspoon dried thyme leaves 1
medium carrot - cut
1 medium stem celery with leaves -- cut up
1 small onion - cut
5 peppercorns
3 whole cloves
3 sprigs parsley
1 dried bay leaf

Heat oil in a 12-to-12-10- to-ice skillet over medium heat. Cook beef in oil until golden on both sides. Mix the rest of the ingredients in a slow 3 1/2 to 6 litre stove. Add beef. Cover and cook over low heat for 8 to 10 hours. Remove beef from broth. Cool beef for about 10 minutes or just until it is cool enough to handle. Strain the two to the other through the sieve lined with cheesecloth; discard vegetables and seasonings. Remove beef from bones. Cut beef into half an inch of beef. Skim the fat from the broth. Use immediately, or cover and refrigerate broth and beef in separate containers for up to 24 hours or freeze for future use.

Yield: About 7 cups Serving size 1 cup Calories 110/Fat 5g/cholesterol 35mg/sodium 460mg carbohydrates 2g/Fiber 1g/Protein 15g

Crockpot beef stew

3 potatoes, diced
5 carrots, diced
4 celery stalks, diced
2 small onions, chopped
1 head (no clove) garlic, finely chopped
1 large tomato, blanched and chopped
4 Tbs. orge
4 cubes of beef stock
1 3/4 pounds lean beef
1/2 tsp rosemary
1/2 tsp salt
1/2 teaspoon
pepper 2 tbsp
flour.
2 Tbs. corn starch

Cube and brown the beef. Add flour to beef and mix. In a saucepan, combine all ingredients except potatoes, corn starch, rosemary and salt. Cover with water. Cook over high heat for 12-24 hours. 1 hour before serving, add potatoes, rosemary and salt. Immediately before serving, thicken with corn starch.

Crockpot beef with mushrooms and red wine sauce

1 1/2 lbs well-stocked beef stew -- cut into 1-inch cubes 2 medium onions
cut into half-inch wedges
1 pkg. champignons sliced fresh mushrooms -- (8 ounces)
1 slice of sturdy onion soup
3 tablespoons cornstarch Salt
and pepper to taste
1 1/2 cups dry red wine

Place beef, onions and mushrooms in a slow cooker of 4 quarters or more (crockpot). Add the dry soup mixture. Sprinkle with cornstarch and salt and pepper to taste. Pour the wine over everything. Cover and cook over low heat for 10 to 12 hours or 5 to 6 hours. Stir well before serving.
6 Portions

Crockpot Big Bowl de Red Chili

3 small onions, chopped
1 chopped green pepper
2 red peppers, chopped
4 garlic cloves, chopped
2 jalapenos -- seeded and chopped
1 large tomato, chopped
56 ounces crushed tomatoes
45 ounces red beans - drained and rinsed
2 tablespoons chili powder
2 tablespoons dried oregano
4 teaspoons cumin
2 teaspoons paprika
4 teaspoons Tabasco sauce
1 teaspoon ground black pepper

Mix all ingredients in a slow cooker. Cook at low setting for 8-10 hours.

Per serving: 343 calories; 3g fat (4% calories from fat); 55g protein; 158g carbohydrates; 0mg Cholesterol; 122mg sodium

Soupe aux haricots noirs Crockpot

8 servings (1 cup)

1/4 lb chorizo
1 small onion, chopped
1 clove garlic, finely chopped
1 small red pepper, chopped
1 small green pepper, chopped
2 tbsp dry sherry
1 tsp ground cumin
1 bay leaf
15 oz   black beans, not angry
15 oz   1 lime FF chicken broth
juice
2 tbsp chopped coriander
1/4 teaspoon salt and pepper

Discard chorizo skin. Crumble the meat and brown in a non-stick frying pan for 2 minutes. Add onion, garlic and peppers. Sauté over medium-high heat for 5 minutes. Add to slow cooker. Add sherry, cumin, bay leaf, beans and broth. Cover and cook over low heat for 4 to 5 hours. Remove the lid. Remove 1 cup of beans and press with the back of a fork to crush. Return to the grass. Add lime juice, coriander, salt and pepper. Simmer uncovered just to warm up, about 5 minutes.

Makes 8 servings (1-cup)

Crockpot Breakfast

32 oz   frozen hash browns
1 lb   cubed ham (lean)
1 diced onion
1 diced green pepper
1 1/2 tbsp grated cheese (ordinary cheese)
12 eggs
1 tsp skimmed milk
1 t salt
1 t black pepper

Divide the potatoes, ham, vegetables and cheese so you can create several layers of each in the slow cooker pot. Start with the hash browns, then the ham, onion peppers and the last cheese. Repeat until you have several layers. Beat eggs, milk salt and pepper pour over layers in slow cooker lid and turn low. Cook for 10 to 12 hours overnight.

12 Portions

Poulet Crockpot

1 10 3/4 oz Can Healthy Demand Cream of Chicken Soup 1 set
dry onion soup mix
2 cups water
2 cups raw instant rice
16 oz skinless, boneless chicken breast, cut into 1-inch pieces 1
cup sliced mushrooms

1/8 tsp black pepper

Spray the slow cooker with cooking spray. In the prepared slow cooker, combine the first 4 ingredients. Add chicken, mushrooms and pepper. Cover and cook over low heat for 6 to 8 hours. Stir before serving. Serves 6 (1 cup)

Crock Pot Chicken #2

4-6 boneless skinless chicken breasts 1/4
tst. white wine
1 pkg. Good season mix of Italian dressing

Brown chicken. Place in slow cooker. Sprinkle dressing mixture over chicken. Add the wine. Cover; cook over high heat for about 4 hours. (Low for 6 - 8 hours.)

Poulet et farce Crockpot

4 chicken breasts (half)
1 pkg. Stove Top Stuffing 1/2
tasse d'eau
1 can of mushroom soup FF cream
1 cup chicken stock

Place chicken on Crockpot stock. Pour broth over chicken. Mix the stuffing, soup and water, and place on top of the chicken. Cook over low heat for 7 hours. Serves 4

Chili au poulet Crockpot

6 skinless chicken thighs
1 large onion - chopped
2 garlic cloves -- finely chopped
1 14.5oz chicken broth
1 teaspoon ground cumin
1 teaspoon dried oregano leaves 1/2
teaspoon salt
1/4 teaspoon red pepper sauce
2 15 oz cans of large northern beans - rinsed and drained 1 15
oz can white shoe ankle corn - drained
3 tablespoons lime juice
2 tablespoons chopped fresh coriander

Remove excess fat from chicken. Combine onion, garlic, broth, cumin, oregano, salt and pepper sauce in a slow cooker of 3 1/2 to 6 litres. Add chicken. Cover and cook over low heat for 4 to 5 hours or until chicken is tender. Remove chicken from slow cooker. Use 2 forks to remove bones and shred chicken into pieces. Discard the bones; return the chicken to the slow cooker. Stir in beans, corn, lime juice and coriander. Cover and cook over low heat for 15 to 20 minutes or until beans and corn are hot.

Per serving: 439 calories; 4g fat; 35g protein; 69g carbohydrates; 22g dietary fibre; 43mg Chl

Fajitas de poulet Crockpot

7 chicken breast halves, boneless and peeled -- cut into strips 2
onions -- sliced
2 green peppers - cut into strips
2 red peppers - cut into strips
2 jalapeno peppers, chopped
4 garlic cloves, chopped
2 teaspoons chili powder
2 teaspoons ground cumin
2 teaspoons ground coriander
28 ounces tomatoes, 1/4 cup
canned water
8 flour tortillas

Mix all ingredients in a slow cooker. Cover and cook over low heat for 8-10 hours. Serve with salsa.

Per serving: 254 calories; 4g fat (15% calories from fat); 23g protein; 32g Carbohydrates; 45mg Cholesterol; 390 mg sodium

Crock Pot Chicken Marengo
Number of servings: 6

Canned sliced mushrooms, drained 10 oz.
Sliced onion 1 cup
Chicken pieces, skin removed 3 lbs.
Canned tomatoes with juice (broken) 14 oz.
Wrap Spaghetti sauce mix 1 x 1-1/2 oz.

Arrange mushrooms and onion in a 5-litre (5-litre) slow cooker. Place chicken pieces on top. Combine tomato and spaghetti sauce in a bowl. Pour over the top of the chicken. Cover. Cook over low heat for 8 to 10 hours or on High for 4 to 5 hours.

Paprika de poulet Crockpot

12 oz chicken breast strips
3 cups potatoes, sliced (skin left optional)
3 cups onions, peeled and sliced
1 cup Pam
Spray Paprika
Water

Place 4 strips on the bottom of the pot. Sprinkle with paprika. Then cover w/ a layer of potatoes. Cover the jars. with a layer of onions. Then spray Pam on it. Then sprinkle generously with paprika. Then start again until you have made 4 layers. Pour the cup of water into the slow cooker (on the side so as not to wash the paprika). Cook high all day and then enjoy.

Soupe tortilla de poulet Crockpot

1 1/2 lbs boneless skinless chicken breasts -- cooked and grated 15 ounces
whole tomatoes
10 elevens enchilada willow
1 medium onion -- chopped
4 ounces chopped green peppers
1 clove garlic - chopped
2 cups water
14 1/2 ounces fat-free chicken broth
1 teaspoon cumin
1 teaspoon chili powder
1 teaspoon salt
1/4 teaspoon ground black pepper 1
whole bay leaf
6 whole corn tortillas
2 tablespoons vegetable oil
1 tablespoon chopped coriander
parmesan cheese -- to garnish

In an electric slow cooker, combine chicken, tomatoes, enchilada sauce, onion, green peppers and garlic. Add water, broth, cumin, chili powder, salt, pepper and bay leaf. Stir in corn. Cover and cook over low heat for 6 to 8 hours or high for 3 to 4 hours. Preheat the oven to 400 degrees. Lightly brush both sides of tortillas with oil. Cut tortillas into 2 1/2 by 1/2-inch strips. Place on a baking sheet. Bake, turning occasionally, until crisp, 5 to 10 minutes. Sprinkle tortilla strips, coriander and parmesan over soup. Makes 6 to 8 servings.

Per serving: 235 calories; 9g Fat; 24g Protein; 16g Carbohydrates; 2g Dietary Fibre; 510mg Sodium.

Soupe tortilla de poulet Crockpot #2

16 Once chicken Breast Halves Without Skin - cubed
30 Ounces black beans, canned -undraded
30 Ounces Mexican-style simmered tomatoes - canned
1 cup Salsa
4 Ounces Chopped Green Peppers
14 1/2 Ounces tomato sauce
2 cups reduced tortilla chips with fatty
cheddar cheese

Combine all ingredients except cheese and tortilla chips in a slow cooker. Cover and cook over low heat for 8 hours. To serve, place a handful of chips in each individual bowl. Ladle soup on chips. Garnish with 1/4 cup of cheese.

Per serving (excluding unknown items): 248 calories; 4g fat (13.2% calories from fat); 25g protein; 27g carbohydrates; 9g dietary fibre; 32mg cholesterol; 1215mg sodium.
Service ideas: Would be good with a spoonful of sour cream too.
 Could also add chopped garlic and coriander to the soup. Could use Monterey Jack cheese instead of Cheddar.

Crock-Pot Chili

1 pound on the round floor
1 cup chopped onion
1/2 cup chopped green pepper 1/4 cup
dry red wine or water
1 tablespoon chili powder
1 teaspoon sugar
1 teaspoon ground cumin
1/4 teaspoon salt
1 clove garlic -- finely chopped
1 15 oz can red beans - drained
1 14.5oz can Mexican-style simmered tomatoes with jalapeno peppers and spices -- nondrained 6 tablespoons of reduced-fat grated extra-point cheddar cheese

Cook the soil in a large non-stick skillet over medium-high heat until brown, stirring to crumble. Add the chopped onion and the following 7 ingredients (garlic onion) and cook for 7 minutes or until the onion is tender. Put the meat mixture in an electric slow cooker and stir in the beans and tomatoes. Cover with lid and cook over low heat for 4 hours. Pour into bowls; sprinkle with cheese. Yield: 6 servings (serving size: 1-1/4 cups chili and 1 tablespoon cheese).

Note: The chilli can be made on the stove if you don't have a slow cooker. After adding the beans and tomatoes, bring to a boil. Reduce heat; simmer, partially covered, for 1-1/2 hours.

NUTRITIONAL INFORMATION: CALORIES 243; FAT 5.6g; PROTEIN 25.5g; CARB 22.9g; FIBER 3.1g; CHOL 49mg; IRON 4.1mg; SODIUM 637mg; CALC 154mg

Crockpot Colorful Chicken Stew

1 lb boneless skinless chicken breasts, cubed
1 (14 1/2 oz) can diced Italian tomatoes, not
2 medium potatoes, peeled and cut into 1/2-inch cubes 5 medium carrots, chopped
3 celery ribs, chopped
1 large onion, chopped
1 medium green pepper, chopped
2 (4 oz) cans of stems and pieces of mushrooms, drained
2 cubes of Low Sodium Artificial Sweetener
Chicken Broth Equal to 2 tsp sugar 1 tsp chili powder
1/4 teaspoon pepper
1 tablespoon cornstarch
2 cups cold water

In a 5-litre slow cooker, combine the first 12 ingredients. In a small bowl, combine cornstarch and water until smooth. Stir in chicken mixture. Cover and cook on LOW for 8 to 10 hours or until vegetables are tender.

Makes 6 servings. Calories.. 123..Fat.. 1 g. Carbohydrates.. 16 g. Protein.. 11g... Sodium... 209 mg ... Fiber... Threeg.

Crockpot Company Chicken Casserole

8 ounces noodles
3 cups boneless skinless chicken breasts -- cooked, diced 1/2 cup
celery -- diced
1/2 cup green pepper -- diced
1/2 cup onion -- diced
4 ounces mushrooms -- canned, drained 1/2
cup un gras chicken stock
1/2 cup fat-free Parmesan cheese
1 can of chicken soup cream -- melted
1 cup pointed cheddar cheese -- grated
1/2 teaspoon basil
1 1/2 cup low-fat cottage cheese - small curd
2 1/2 cups water

Cook the noodles according to the package instructions until they are barely tender; drain and rinse well. In a large bowl, mix remaining ingredients with noodles, making sure noodles are separated and covered with liquid. Pour the mixture into a greased slow cooker. Cover and cook on LOW for 6-10 hours. Can cook on HIGH for 3-4 hours.

Per serving: 467.3 cal.11.7 g (23.4%) fat, 1.7g fibre, 824 mg sodium

Fettuccine de poulet crémeux Crockpot

1 1/2 pounds boneless skinless chicken breasts -- cubed 1/2 teaspoon
garlic powder
1/2 teaspoon onion powder
1/8 teaspoon pepper
1 10-3/4 ounce condensed cream of chicken soup - undiluted 1 10-3/4
ounces can condensed celery soup cream - undiluted 4 ounces Of
American cheese process - cubed
1 2-1/4 ounces sliced ripe olives - drained
1 2-ounce jar diced pimientos - drained, optional
1 16 ounces packing of spinach fettuccine or spaghetti thin
baguettes - optional

Place chicken in slow cooker; sprinkle with garlic powder, onion powder and pepper. Garnish with soups. Cover and cook over high heat for 3 to 4 hours or until chicken juice is clear. Stir in cheese, olives and pimientos if desired. Cover and cook until cheese is melted. Meanwhile, cook the fettuccine according to the instructions of the package; Aspire. Serve with chicken and chopsticks if desired.

Makes 6 servings. Calories... 210...Fat... 7.1g... Carbohydrates... 8g... Protein... 26g... Sodium... 856 mg... Fiber... 0.2 g.

Sandwiches Crockpot Easy English Dip

3 pounds fresh beef breast (no corned beef)
1 1.3 oz dry onion soup mixture
1 10.5 oz condensed beef stock
8 mini baguettes or sandwich buns

Place beef in a slow cooker of 3 1/2 to 6 litres. Combine dry soup mixture and beef broth; pour over the beef. Cover and cook over low heat for 8 to 10 hours or until beef is tender. Skim the fat from the liquid.

Remove beef; cut through the grain into thin slices. Cut each baguette horizontally in half. Fill beef chopsticks; bœuf; cut in half. Serve with broth for dipping.

Makes 8 sandwiches 1 sandwich 270 calories Fat 10g/Cholesterol 60mg/Sodium 20mg/Carbohydrates 20g/Fiber 1g/protein 26g

Favorite pot roast of the Crockpot family

2 1/2 pounds round roast beef stock
2 teaspoons olive or vegetable oil
3 medium potatoes -- cut into 2-inch pieces
2 1/2 cups carrots cut by baby
2 cups sliced mushrooms
1 medium-stemmed celery -- sliced
1 medium onion -- chopped
1 teaspoon salt
1/2 teaspoon pepper
1/2 teaspoon dried thyme leaves
1 14.5 oz   diced tomatoes -- not
1 10.5 oz can condensed consumed beef or broth
1 5.5 oz   juice of eight vegetables 1/4
cup Gold Medal all-purpose flour

Remove excess fat from beef. Heat oil in 10-inch skillet over medium-high heat. Cook beef in oil for about 10 minutes, turning occasionally; until it is brown on all sides. Place potatoes, carrots, mushrooms, celery and onion in a slow 4 to 5 litre pan. Sprinkle with salt, pepper and thyme. Place beef on top of vegetables. Pour tomatoes, consumed and vegetable juice over beef.

Cover and cook over low heat for 8 to 10 hours or until beef and vegetables are tender. Remove beef and vegetables from slow cooker with a slotted spoon; place on the serving tray and keep warm. Cut the fat from beef juice in the slow cooker if desired. Remove one-and-a-half cup of juice from the slow cooker; mix with flour until smooth with a metal whisk. Gradually add the flour mixture to the remaining juice in a slow cooker. Cook over high heat for about 15 minutes or until thickened. Serve sauce with beef and vegetables.

Nutrition Information: 1 serving 255 calories Fat 6g/Cholesterol 75mg/Sofium 880mg/Carbohydrates 24g/Fiber 4g/Protein 32g

Crockpot Green Chili Chicken Stew

5 chicken breast halves, boneless and peeled whole -- cut into 1 1/4
teaspoons ground cumin cubes
1 teaspoon dried sage
2 large onions -- chopped
2 garlic cloves -- finely chopped
1 tablespoon cider vinegar
6 Small red potatoes -- in wedges
3 whole poblano peppers - seeded and diced
10 tomatillos - inked, chopped
1 1/2 cups fat-free chicken broth 1/2
cup chopped coriander

The original recipe called for 2 pounds of round beef or chuck, cut into 1 inch pieces, but I replaced 5 boneless, skinless chicken breast halves, and it turned out fine. Mix all ingredients except coriander in slow cooker. Cover and cook at low setting for 8-10 hours. Serve garnished with chopped coriander.

Per serving: 220 calories; 2g fat; 29g protein; 24g carbohydrates; 4g dietary fibre; 57mg cholesterol; 199mg sodium.

Crockpot Ham et Lima Beans

1 pound dried Lima beans - soaked overnight
1 whole onion, chopped
1 whole green pepper - chopped
1 teaspoon dry mustard
1 teaspoon salt
1 teaspoon pepper
1/4 pound extra lean ham or bacon (up to 1/2 lb) - cut into small pieces 1 cup
water
1 can of tomato soup

Put all the ingredients in the crock-pot. Stir well. Cover and cook over low heat for 7 to 10 hours, 4 to 5 hours. Can be served with hot cornbread.

Per serving: 309 calories; 2g fat; 21g protein; 54g carbohydrates; 15g dietary fibre; 9mg Cholesterol; 757mg sodium.

Crockpot Home-Style Turkey Dinner

3 medium Yukon golden potatoes - cut into 2-inch pieces
3 turkey legs -- skin removed
1 12 oz homemade pot style turkey sauce
2 tablespoons of all-purpose Gold Medal flour
1 teaspoon parsley flakes
1/2 teaspoon dried thyme leaves 1/8
teaspoon pepper
1 1lb frozen bag of beans and carrots mixture - thawed and drained

Place potatoes in a slow 3 1/2 to 6 litre stove; place the turkey on top. Mix remaining ingredients except vegetables until smooth; pour over the mixture in a slow cooker. Cover and cook over low heat for 8 to 10 hours or until turkey juice is no longer pink when the thickest parts centres are cut. Stir in vegetables.

Cover and cook over low heat for about 30 minutes or until vegetables are tender. Remove turkey and vegetables from slow cooker with a slotted spoon. Mix the sauce; serve with turkey and vegetables.

Nutrition Information: 1 Portion 335 calories Fat 8g/Cholesterol 155mg/Sodium/450 mg/Carbohydrates 26g/Fiber 4g/protein 44g

Poulet italien Crockpot

4 whole boneless skinless chicken breast Half 16 ounces
tomatoes - (or 2-3 fresh tomatoes)
1 whole onion - sliced
1 teaspoon Italian seasoning
1 whole green bell pepper -- salted and chopped salt and
pepper -- to taste

Throw everything in the slow cooker and cook at about 8-10 hours.

Per serving: 171 calories; 2g total fat; 29g protein; 9g carbohydrates; 68mg Cholesterol; 88mg sodium

Crockpot #2 de poulet italien

portions: 12

3lb boneless frozen, skinless chicken breast (thawed)
1 envelope Good Seasons Italian Dressing (dry not made) I used their low fat envelope an
envelope 1 Onion soup mix (dry not made)
1 tsp minced garlic or garlic (I used fresh)
1 sweet or hot pepperoncini jar (your choice)

Put all the chicken in a slow cooker sprayed with Pam. In a bowl, mix the rest of the ingredients (with pepperoncini juice and all) together, taking care not to break the peppers. Pour over chicken and cook for 8 to 9 hours over low heat. No glance. Once done, choose the peppers and put in a serving dish to use on sandwiches for those who like warmer sandwiches. Using a sturdy spoon break the chicken, it is very very tender. Serve 1/2 cup on a healthy Lite bread. Drain most of the juices, add the BBQ sauce for the excellent BBQ sandwiches the next day. Freeze in small containers to have in a pinch.

Poulet au citron Crockpot

6 skinless skinless chicken breasts without skin
1/2 cup all-purpose flour
1 teaspoon salt
1 tablespoon balsamic vinegar
3 tablespoons ketchup
3 tablespoons brown sugar
6 oz   frozen lemonade concentrate
2 tablespoons corn water
1/4 cup water

Dredge the chicken in flour mixed with salt. Shake the excess and brown in a hot frying pan. Remove chicken and place in slow cooker. Mix lemonade, brown sugar, vinegar (use plain vinegar if you prefer) and catsup and pour over chicken. Cook over high heat for 3-4 hours. Once ready to serve, remove chicken on a hot tray and thicken sauce with cornstarch/water solution, and serve with chicken.

Per serving: 384 calories; 3g fat; 56g protein; 30g carbohydrates; 1g dietary fibre; 137mg Cholesterol; 601mg sodium.

Crockpot Meatloaf Recipe

l LB extra lean ground beef 1
LB ground turkey
2 cups soft breadcrumbs 1/2
cup Marinara sauce 1 whole
egg
2 tablespoons dried onion - chopped
1 1/4 teaspoons salt
1 teaspoon garlic salt
1/2 teaspoon dried Italianseasoning.. crushed 1/4
teaspoon garlic powder
1/4 teaspoon pepper
2 tablespoons Marinara sauce

Fold a 30-inch-long piece of aluminum foil in half lengthwise. Place at the bottom of a slow cooker with both ends hanging on the top edge of the stove. In a large bowl, combine ground beef, ground turkey, breadcrumbs, 1/2 cup marinara sauce, egg, onion, salt, garlic salt, Italian herbs, garlic powder and pepper until well blended. Shape yourself into bread. Place in slow cooker on top of foil. Spread 2 tablespoons of marinara sauce on top. Cover tightly and cook on LOW for 5 to 6 hours or on HIGH for 2 1/2 to 3 hours. Use the ends of the foil to lift the meatloaf and transfer to a serving dish.

Yield: 8 slices per serving: 271 calories(kcal); 16g Total Fat

Mexican Pig Crockpot

1 pound boneless pork loin roast - cut into 1 20 oz   pot
salsa pieces
1 4 oz can chopped green peppers - drained
1 15 oz can black beans - rinsed and drained
1 cup grated Monterey jack cheese - if desired

Combine pork, salsa and chillies in a slow 3 1/2 to 4 litre cooker. Cover and cook over low heat for 6 to 8 hours or until pork is tender. Stir in beans. Cover and cook for about 5 minutes or until hot. Sprinkle with cheese.

1 serving 345 calories/Fat 10g/Cholesterol 75mg/Sodium 900 mg/Carbohydrates 37g/Fiber 10g/Protein 37g

Soupe multi-haricots Crockpot

5 14.5 oz chicken or vegetable broth
1 20 oz 15 or 16 bean soup mixtures - sorted and rinsed 4 medium carrots
- chopped
3 medium celery stalks -- chopped
1 large onion - chopped
2 tablespoons tomato paste
1 teaspoon salt
1 teaspoon Italian seasoning 1/2
teaspoon pepper
1 14.5oz can be diced tomatoes - drained

Mix all ingredients except tomatoes in a 5 to 6 litre slow cooker. Cover and cook over low heat for 8 to 10 hours or until beans are tender. Stir in tomatoes. Cover and cook over high heat for about 15 minutes or until hot.

Per serving: 25 calories; fat trace; 1 g protein; 6g carbohydrates; 2g dietary fiber; 0mg Cholesterol; 220mg sodium.

Crockpot Pork Chop Supper

6 pork chops - 1/2 inch thick
6 medium new potatoes -- cut into eighths
1 10.75 oz   cream condensed mushroom soup
1 4 oz can pieces of mushrooms and stems - drained
2 tablespoons dry white wine 1/4
teaspoon dried thyme leaves 1/2
teaspoon garlic powder
1/2 teaspoon Worcestershire sauce
3 tablespoons Gold Medal all-purpose flour
1 tablespoon diced pimientos
1 10 oz 10 oz frozen green peas -- rinsed and drained

Spray the 10-inch non-stick skillet with a cooking spray; heat over medium-high heat. Cook the pork in the pan, turning once, until golden. Place potatoes in a slow 3 1/2 to 6 litre stove. Combine soup, mushrooms, wine, thyme, garlic powder, Worcestershire sauce and flour; spoon half of the soup mixture over the potatoes. Place pork on top of potatoes, cover with remaining soup mixture. Cover and cook over low heat for 6 to 7 hours or until pork is tender. Remove pork; keep warm. Stir the pimientos and peas into a slow cooker. Cover and cook over low heat for about 15 minutes or until peas are tender. Serve with pork.

1 serving 275 calories/fats 11g/cholesterol 65mg/sodium 520mg/carbohydrate 21g/fibre 4g/protein 27g

Chowder de pommes de terre Crockpot
8 servings (1 1/4 cups)

2 cups potatoes, cut into 1/2-inch cubes
1 large carrot, diced
1 cup chopped leek, only white part
1 clove garlic, finely chopped
4 cups fat-free chicken broth 1/2
cup pearl barley
1 bay leaf
1/4 teaspoon dried thyme and
crushed 1/4 teaspoon pepper.
4 oz Canadian bacon. cut into half-inch pieces 1/2
cup of evaporated fat-free milk
1/4 cup fat-free half-and-half

In a slow cooker, combine potatoes, carrots, leek, garlic, chicken broth, barley, bay leaf, thyme, pepper and Canadian bacon. Cover and cook over low heat for 6 hours or until vegetables and barley are tender. Stir in the evaporated milk and half and heat through, uncovered, about 10 minutes.

Makes 8 servings (1 1/4 cups)

Pork fajitas from Crockpot

1 2 1/2 pound boneless pork loin roast
1 medium onion -- thinly sliced
2 cups barbecue sauce 3/4
cup salsa
3 tablespoons chili powder
1 tablespoon Mexican seasoning
9 flour tortillas

Remove excess fat from pork. Place pork in a slow 3 1/2 to 6 litre stove; arrange the onion on top. Mix remaining ingredients except tortillas; pour over the pork. Cover and cook over low heat for 8 to 10 hours or until pork is very tender. Remove pork; place on a large plate. Use 2 forks to pull the pig to shreds. Pour the sauce into a bowl; stir in pork. Pour filling over tortillas; roll.

1 serving 395 calories/fats 15g/cholesterol 80mg/sodium 790mg/carbohydrate 35g/fibre 4g/protein 34g

Poulet et légumes Crockpot Savory

8 boneless, skinless chicken thighs
2 cups chicken broth
1 teaspoon salt
1/4 teaspoon pepper 8
ounces pearl onions
6 slices bacon - cooked and crumbled
2 cloves garlic - finely chopped
Bouquet Garni - See below
1 bag of carrots, cut by baby
1 pound of small mushrooms with whole buttons
2 tablespoons Gold Medal all-purpose flour
2 tablespoons cold water

Place chicken in a 5 to 6 litre slow cooker. Add remaining ingredients except mushrooms, flour and water. Cover and cook over low heat for 8 to 10 hours or until chicken juice is no longer pink when the thickest pieces are cut. Remove any grease from the surface. Remove Bouquet Garni. Stir in mushrooms. Mix flour and water; stir in chicken mixture. Cover and cook over high heat for 30 minutes or until thickened.

For Bouquet Garni: Attach 4 sprigs of parsley, 2 bay leaves and 1 teaspoon of dried thyme leaves in a cheesecloth bag or place them in a tea ball.

Per serving: 46 calories; 3g fat; 3g protein; 2g carbohydrates; dietary fibre trace; 4mg Cholesterol; 601mg sodium.

Soupe Crockpot

1 whole green pepper - (or red), chopped
1 whole onion - chopped
16 ounces ground beef sirloin (90/10)
14 1/2 ounces chicken broth, Swanson, 100% fat-free
15 1/2 ounces pinto beans, canned
15 ounces corn, canned
15 ounces pork and beans
1 ounce chili seasoning mixture -- (1 pkg.)
29 ounces tomatoes, canned -- (2 cans), chopped
3 ounces elbow macaroni -- dry weight

Spray the Dutch oven with Pam ground beef. Brown, green pepper and onion. Add all other ingredients except macaroni. Simmer (or cook in a slow cooker) until flavours blend well. 20 minutes before serving, add the macaroni of the elbow. Cook until macaroni is tender.

Serves 8 (1 3/8 cup each).
344 cal, 8 g fat, 8 g fiber, 21 g prot, 45 g carbohydrates, 893 mg turf, 87 mg calc

Crock #1 pot soup

1 can chicken broth
1 onion, chopped
1 red pepper
1 can pinto beans
1 can of drained corn
1 can of pork and beans
1 mix of packaged chili seasoning
2 cans chopped tomatoes

Put all the ingredients in the slow cooker and simmer all day. Each serving: 1 1/2 C.

Chicken salsa with Crockpot sour cream

4 skinless boneless chicken breast halves
1 low-sodium taco seasoning package
1 cup salsa
2 tablespoons cornstarch 1/4
cup light sour cream

Spray the slow cooker with cooking spray. Add chicken breasts. Sprinkle with Taco seasoning. Garnish with salsa. Cook over low heat for 6-8 hours. When ready to serve, remove the chicken from the pan. Place about 2 tablespoons of cornstarch in a small amount of water. Stir well. Stir the cornstarch mixture into the salsa sauce. Stir in 1/4 cup sour cream.

Per serving: 170 calories; 2g fat; 28g protein; 9g carbohydrates; 1g dietary fibre; 70mg cholesterol; 403mg sodium

Crockpot Split Split Pea Soup

2 1/2 cups split peas
1 1/2 cups extra lean ham - diced
1 tablespoon reduced-calorie margarine
1 tablespoon oil
2 whole carrots - peeled and diced
1 medium potato - peeled and diced
1 whole onion - diced
4 cups water
2 cups fat-free chicken broth
with salt and pepper flavour

Sauté the diced onion in butter and oil until golden. Place onion and remaining ingredients in slow cooker, cover, cook over medium heat for 8-10 hours. The time may be slightly longer at higher altitudes. Per serving: 392 calories; 6g fat; 31g protein; 58g carbohydrates; 22g dietary fibre; 16mg Cholesterol

Steak suisse Crockpot

3 tablespoons Gold Medal all-purpose flour
1 teaspoon ground mustard
1/2 teaspoon salt
1 1/2 pounds round boneless beef, tip or chuck steak - cut into 6 pieces 2
tablespoons vegetable oil
1 large onion - sliced
1 large pepper -- sliced
1 14.5oz can diced tomatoes - nondrained
2 garlic cloves -- finely chopped

Combine flour, mustard and salt. Coat beef with flour mixture. Heat oil in a 10-inch skillet over medium heat. Cook beef in oil for about 15 minutes, turning once, until golden. Place beef in a slow cookery of 3 1/2 to 6 litres; garnish with onion and pepper. Mix tomatoes and garlic; pour over beef and vegetables. Cover and cook over low heat for 7 to 9 hours or until beef is tender.

1 serving 190 calories Fat 7g/Cholesterol 60mg/Sodium 340mg/Carbohydrates 10g/Fiber 2g/protein 24g

Crockpot Tuscan Pasta

1 pound boneless skinless chicken breast - cut into 1" 15 ounces of red
beans, canned - rinsed and drained
15 ounces canned tomato sauce
29 ounces Italian-style tomatoes - simmered, 2 - 14 1/2 ounces cans of
mushrooms 4 1/2 ounces of mushrooms, canned - drained
1 medium green pepper - 1/2 cup chopped
onion
1/2 cup chopped celery 4
cloves garlic - chopped 1
cup water
1 teaspoon dried Italian seasoning
6 ounces spaghetti - thin, uncooked, broken in half

Place all ingredients except spaghetti in slow cooker. Cover and cook over low heat for 4 hours or until vegetables are tender. Turn up. Stir in spaghetti; Cover. Stir again after 10 minutes. Cover and cook for 45 minutes, or until pasta is tender.

Per serving: 247 Calories); (kcal); 1 g total fat; 21g protein; 37g carbohydrates; 33mg Cholesterol; 843mg Sodium 7 grams fiber

CrockPot Vegetable Pasta

2 teaspoons margarine
1 zucchini -- 1/4-inch slice
1 yellow squash -- 1/4-inch slice
2 carrots -- thinly sliced
1 1/2 cups mushrooms -- fresh, sliced
1 packet broccoli - cuts
4 sliced green onions
1 clove of garlic, chopped
1/2 teaspoon basil - dried
1/4 teaspoon salt
1/2 teaspoon pepper
1 cup grated Parmesan cheese
12 ounces fettucine
1 cup en low-fat mozzarella cheese
1 cup of low-fat milk
2 Egg

Rub the slow cooker wall with butter. Place zucchini, yellow squash, carrots, mushrooms, broccoli, onions, garlic, seasonings and parmesan in the pot of simmer. Cover; cook on High 2 hours. Cook fettucine according to package instructions; drain. Add la fettucinecuite,mozzarella, cream and egg yolks. Stir to mix well. Heat for 15 to 30 minutes. To serve, turn to Low for up to 30 minutes. Serves six.

Per serving: 431 calories; 12g fat (25% calories from fat); 23g protein; 58g carbohydrates; 95mg Cholesterol; 493 mg sodium

Cuban black beans

1 pound dried black beans - sorted and rinsed
1 cup onion -- chopped (1 large)
1 1/2 cups pepper -- chopped (1 large)
5 garlic cloves -- finely chopped
14 1/2 ounces diced tomatoes --unsrained (1 can)
5 cups water
2 tablespoons olive oil -- (or vegetable oil)
4 teaspoons ground cumin
2 teaspoons jalapeno chile pepper - finely chopped
1 teaspoon salt
2 bay leaves, whole

Mix all ingredients in a slow cooker. Cook over high heat for 6-8 hours. Remove bay leaves before serving. Serve over hot cooked rice. Garnish with diced hard-boiled eggs, hot sauce and/or diced red onion.

Per serving: 341 calories; 6g total fat; 18g protein; 57g carbohydrates; 0mg Cholesterol; 375mg sodium

Drunk rosemary chicken with basmati rice

FACT: 4 to 6 servings

8 chicken thighs (23/4 to 3 lbs in total)
Salt and freshly ground pepper
6 garlic cloves, peeled and thinly sliced
1 teaspoon coarsely chopped fresh rosemary leaves or dried rosemary 1 cup
Chardonnay or other dry white wines
1/2 cup skimmed chicken broth 1 1/2 cups
pre-cooked dried white rice
1/4 cup chopped green onions (including tops)
rosemary sprigs, rinsed

Rinse the thighs and dry. Remove and discard skin; cut and discard the pieces of grease. Lightly sprinkle the thighs with salt and pepper. Place the thighs in a 41/2-quarter or more electric slow-cooker. Sprinkle with garlic and chopped rosemary; haché; pour the wine and broth over the chicken. Cover and cook until meat pulls easily from bone, about 5 hours over low heat, 3 hours high. Cut and discard the fat from the juices. Add rice and mix to moisten evenly. Turn the stove to high; cover and cook, stirring several times, until rice is tender to bite, about 5 minutes. Pour chicken and rice onto a platter. Sprinkle with onions and garnish with sprigs of rosemary. Add salt and pepper to taste.

Per serving: 242 cal., 17% (42 cal.) fat; 26 g protein; 4.7 g fat (1.2 g sat.); 21 g carbo (0.6 g fiber); 113 mg sodium; 99 mg chol.

Easiest Crock Pot Chicken

1 Packet chicken breast halves
1 Can 98% fat-free cream of mushroom soup 1 Can
98% fat-free cream of chicken soup

Skin chicken pieces (or use boneless, skinless chicken breasts). Place in slow cooker. Mix the soups and pour over the chicken. Cook over low heat all day. Remove chicken from sauce - remove bones. Serve over hot rice.

Per serving: 62 calories; 3g fat; 8g protein; trace carbohydrates; trace of dietary fiber; 23mg Cholesterol; 26mg sodium.

Easy baked beans

2 cans (28 oz each) vegetarian baked beans, drained
1 m onion, chopped (1/2 cup) 2/3
cup barbecue sauce
1/2 cup brown sugar packaged
2 tbsp ground mustard (dry)

Mix all ingredients in a slow cookery of 3 1/2 to 6 qt. Cover and cook on LOW for 4 to 5 hours. (orou HIGH 2 2 1/2 hours.) or until desired consistency. Per serving: cal 190, fat 1g, sat fat 0g, chol 0mg, turf 940mg, carbohydrates 43g, fiber 8g, prot 10g Made 10 servings

Easy cassoulet

8 ounces boneless skinless chicken thighs
2 medium carrots -- cut into 1/2-inch pieces
1 medium red or green sweet pepper -- cut into one-and-a-half-
inch pieces 1 cup onions -- chopped
3 garlic cloves -- finely chopped
30 ounces white or northern beans - rinsed and drained 14 1/2 ounces Italian-
style simmered tomatoes - not
8 ounces smoked turkey sausage, fully cooked - halved lengthwise and --cut into 1/2" slices 1 1/2
cups dry white wine or chicken broth
1 tablespoon parsley, fresh - cut
1 teaspoon thyme, dried - crushed 1/4
teaspoon ground red pepper
1 bay leaf

Rinse chicken; pat it down. Cut chicken into 1-inch pieces. Place carrots, pepper, onion, garlic, beans, tomatoes, chicken and sausages in a 3 1/2, 4 or 5-quarter dish cooker. In a bowl, combine chicken broth or wine, parsley, thyme, red pepper and bay leaf. Add to the dishtop. Cover and cook over low heat for 7 to 8 hours or over high heat for 3 and a half to 4 hours. Discard the bay leaf. Per serving: 259 cals; 7 g total fat; 44 mg chol;974 mg sodium; 31 g carbohydrates; 8 g dietary fiber; cals

Easy Hearty Turkey Chili

Yield: 6-1 Portion Cups

1 Large onion
2 cloves garlic
1/2 Lb Ground Turkey
2 Tbs. Chili Powder
1 Tbs. Paprika
1 Tsp. Ground Cumin
2 Tbs. Crushed cherry peppers
2 tomatoes, chopped
1 cup fat-free chicken broth
1 1/2 tbsp cider vinegar
2 cups red beans
1 Bell Green Pepper

I throw it all in a pot of slow cooker and cook for 2 hours over high heat or 4 hours over low heat. It's a delicious meal; 1 cup is very filling, especially if you eat it with baked tortilla chips. Enjoy it.

Easy Italian vegetable soup

14 1/2 ounces diced tomatoes --unsrained (1 can)
10 1/2 ounces condensed beef stock -- undiluted (1 can) 8
ounces sliced mushrooms
1 medium zucchini -- thinly sliced
1 medium green pepper, chopped
1 medium yellow onion, chopped
1/3 cup dry red wine - OR 1/3 cup beef stock 1 1/2
tablespoons dried basil leaves
2 1/2 teaspoons sugar
1 tablespoon extra virgin olive oil 1/2
teaspoon extra virgin salt
4 ounces shredded mozzarella cheese -- (1 cup), optional

In a slow cooker, combine tomatoes, broth, mushrooms, zucchini, pepper, onion, wine, basil and sugar. Cook on LOW 8 hours or on HIGH 4 hours. Stir oil and salt into soup. Garnish with cheese, if desired. Makes 5 to 6 servings.

Per serving: 92 calories; 3g fat; 4g protein; 12g carbohydrates; 3g dietary fibre; 0mg Cholesterol; 454mg sodium.

Eight-layer casserole
Makes 4-5 servings

1/2 lb lean ground beef
2 tbsp imitation bacon pieces
1 small onion, chopped
1 (15 oz) can tomato sauce 1/2
cup water
1/2 teaspoon chili
powder 1/4 teaspoon
salt
1/4 teaspoon ground black
pepper 2/3 cup long grain rice
1 (8 3/4 oz) whole grain corn, drained 1/2 cup
chopped green pepper

Crumble the beef evenly on the bottom of a slow 3 1/2 qt stove. Sprinkle with bacon pieces, then onion. In a med bowl. pour half over the layers of beef and onion. Sprinkle rice evenly on top, then corn. Garnish with remaining tomato sauce mixture, then bell pepper. Cover and cook on LOW for about 5 hours. or until the rice is tender.

Per serving: 365 cal, 47g carbohydrates, 16g prot,,13g fat, 5g sat fat, sat42mg chol,1071mg turf

Favorite family Chile

Makes 8 servings

2 lbs ground beef
1 large onion, chopped (1 cup)
2 garlic cloves, finely chopped
1 can (28 oz) diced tomatoes, not
11 cans (15 oz) tomato sauce
2 tbsp chili powder
1 1/2 teaspoons ground
cumin 1/2 teaspoon salt
1/2 teaspoon pepper
1 can (15 or 16 oz) kidney or pinto beans, rinsed and drained

Cook beef in a 12-inch skillet over med heat. Aspire. Mix the beef and the rest of the ingredients, except the beans, in a slow cookery of 3 1/2 to 6 qt.. Cover and cook on LOW 6 to 8 hours. (orou HIGH 3 to 4 hours.) or until the onion is tender. Stir in beans. Cover and cook on HIGH for 15 to 20 minutes or until slightly thickened.

Per serving: cal 335, fat 17g, fat sat 7g, chol 65mg, turf 820mg, carbohydrates 24g, fiber 6g, prot 28g

Forgotten Minestrone

1 pound round steak -- cut into 2-inch pieces, lean
6 cups water
1 28 oz   canned tomatoes -- cut, sliced 2 cubes of beef
stock
1 medium onion, chopped
2 tablespoons dried parsley 1/2
teaspoon salt - optional 1 1/2
teaspoons thyme
1/2 teaspoon pepper
1 medium zucchini -- thinly sliced
1 16 oz 1 16 oz garbanzo beans -- rinsed and drained
1 cup elbow macaroni -- or small shells
1/4 cup optional grated Parmesan cheese

In a slow cooker, combine beef, water, tomatoes, broth, onion, parsley, salt if desired, thyme and pepper. Cover and cook over low heat for 7 to 9 hours or until meat is tender. Add zucchini, cabbage, beans and macaroni; cook over high heat, covered, 30-45 minutes more, or until vegetables are tender. Sprinkle individual portions with Parmesan cheese if desired.

Frankfurters avec Macaroni et Fromage

4 cups elbow-cooked macaroni, rinsed and drained
1 1/2 cups (1 12 liquid once can) Evaporated skimmed milk of ametic 1
cup skimmed milk
2 tablespoons dried onion flakes
1 teaspoon dried parsley flakes
2 cups (8 ounces) grated Kraft reduced-fat cheddar cheese 8 ounces
Healthy Choice 97 percent fat-free frankfurters, diced

Combine macaroni, evaporated skim milk, skimmed milk, onion flakes and parsley flakes in a slow cooker spray flavoured with butter. Add cheddar cheese and frankfurters. Mix well to combine. Cover and cook over low heat for 3 to 4 hours. Mix well before serving.
Serves 8 (1 cup).

Each serving is equivalent to: 246 calories, 6 grams of fat, 18 grams of protein, 30 grams of carbohydrates, 525 milligrams of sodium, 371 milligrams of calcium and 1 gram of fiber.

Roast pork with garlic

3 1/2 pounds boneless pork loin roast
1 tablespoon vegetable oil
1 teaspoon salt
1/2 teaspoon pepper
1 medium onion -- sliced
3 garlic cloves -- peeled
1 cup fat-free chicken broth or water

Cut off excess pork fat. heat oil in a 10-inch skillet over medium-high heat. cook pork in oil for about 10 minutes, turning occasionally, until golden on all sides. Sprinkle with salt and pepper. Place onion and garlic in a slow 3 1/2 to 6 litre stove. Place pork on onion and garlic. Pour broth over pork. Cover and cook over low heat for 8-10 hours or until pork is tender.
Per serving; 203 Calories; 8g fat; 30g protein; 1g carbohydrate; dietary fibre trace; 72mg Cholesterol; 322mg sodium.

Glow pork chops

5 whole pork loin chops -- (5 to 6) 1/4
cup brown sugar
1/2 tsp ground cinnamon 1/4
teaspoon ground cloves
8 ounces tomato sauce
29 ounces cling peach halves 1/4
cup vinegar
to taste Salt and pepper

Slightly golden pork axes on both sides. Pour in the excess fat. Combine sugar, cinnamon, cloves, tomato sauce, 1/4 cup peach syrup and vinegar. Sprinkle chops with salt and pepper. Arrange chops in a slow cooker. Place drained peach halves on top. Pour the tomato mixture into the mixture. Cover and cook for 4 to 6 hours.

5-6 servings per serving: 176 calories; 4g fat; 17g protein; 18g carbohydrates; 2g dietary fibre; 39mg cholesterol; 268mg sodium.

Ginger pork wraps

3 tbsp grated ginger
3 tbsp honey
2 1/2 pounds roasted boneless pork loin - adorned with fat
1/4 cup hosin sauce
3 cups bought coleslaw mixture
2 tbsp rice vinegar
12 flour tortillas without whole fats -- (8-10") heated

In 3 slow cookers of 1/2 to 4 qt, mix ginger root and honey; mix well. Add the roast pork; turn to coat with honey mixture. Cover; cook at low setting for 6-8 hours. Remove the roast from the slow cooker. With 2 forks, tattered pork; lambeaux; back to the slow cooker. Stir in hoisin sauce. In the med bowl. mix well. To serve, spread about 1/3 cup of pork mixture in the center of each hot tortilla. Garnish each with a cabbage salad mixture of one to four cups. Roll each closely.

12 sandwiches per serving: 242 calories; 10g fat; 16g protein; 22g carbohydrates; 6g dietary fibre; 49mg Cholesterol; 291mg sodium.

Ham and potatoes with Gratin

2 cups, diced extra-lean ham
4 cups diced raw potatoes
1 cup chopped onion
3/4 cup reduced-fat grated cheddar cheese 1 (10 3/4 ounces) can be healthy in demand
Celery soup cream 1/8
tsp black pepper
1 tsp dried parsley flakes
1 tsp prepared yellow mustard

Spray a slow cooker with butter-flavoured cooking spray. Combine ham, potatoes and onion. Sprinkle cheddar cheese evenly on top. In a small bowl, combine celery soup, black pepper, parsley flakes and mustard. Add soup mixture to potato mixture. Mix well to combine. Cover and cook on LOW for 8 hours. Mix well before serving.

Makes 6 (1 cup) 181 calories, 5 gam Fat,3 gm Fiber

Burger and noodle soup

Makes 6 servings (1 1/3 cups)

1 lb lean or extra-lean ground beef
1 med. onion, coarsely chopped
1 stem celery, cut into 1/4-inch slices
1)1.15 oz.) pkg. mélange dry mixture of strong mushroom soup
1 (14.5 oz) diced tomatoes, not
3 cups water 1/2
teaspoon salt 1/4
teaspoon.
2 cups frozen, thawed and drained mixed vegetables
2 oz (1 cup) uncooked fine egg noodles

Brown ground beef in a large frying pan until cooked through, stirring frequently. Drain well. In 4-6 qt. slow cooker, mix cooked ground beef with all remaining ingredients except mixed vegetables and noodles; mix well. Cover; cook on LOW for 6-8 hours.

About 20 minutes before serving, add thawed vegetables and egg noodles to soup; mix well. Increase heat setting to HIGH; cover and cook for an additional 15-20 minutes or until vegetables are tender and noodles are tender.

Per serving: Cal 260, fat 11g, sat fat 4 g, chol 55 mg, turf 720 mg, carbohydrates 22g, fib 3g, prot 17g

Potluck Ham Cook

1 1/2 cups grated carrots
6 cups (20oz) grated frozen potatoes
9 oz (full1/2 cup) Diced Dubuque 97% fat-free ham or any extra-lean 1 tablespoon dried onion flakes
1 (10 3/4 oz) can Healthy Demand Cream of Mushroom Soup 1/4 cup skimmed milk
1/8 teaspoon black pepper
3/4 cup (3oz) grated Kraft Cheddar Cheese

In a slow cooker container, combine carrots, potatoes, ham and onion flakes. Add mushroom soup, skim milk, black pepper and cheddar cheese. Mix well to combine. Cover and cook on LOW for 6 to 8 hours. Stir well before serving. Divide into 6 servings.

Hearty Italian spaghetti dinner

12 ounces pork loin, lean, boneless -- cut with fat, cut into 1x 1/4-inch (4-4 oz) strips 1 cup onion -- finely chopped
1/2 cup sun-dried tomatoes -- cut 1 tablespoon dried parsley
1 tablespoon dried Italian seasoning 1/2 teaspoon salt
4 garlic cloves -- finely chopped
28 ounces crushed tomatoes -- mashed, non-designed (1 can) 8 ounces tomato sauce -- (1 can)
12 ounces spaghetti - uncooked

In 3-1/2 or 4-quarter Crock-Pot Slow Cooker, combine all ingredients except spaghetti; mix well. Cover; cook at low setting for at least 7 hours or until pork is no longer pink and onions are tender. Cook spaghetti at the desired cooking time as indicated on the package. Aspire. Serve pork mixture over spaghetti.

6 servings per serving: 356 calories; 4g fat; 21g protein; 60g carbohydrates; 6g dietary fibre; 26mg Cholesterol; 696mg sodium.

Hearty meatball chowder

1 cup serving Size: 12

1 cup water
2 cans of tomato soup
1 1/2 cups potatoes - diced
1 can diced tomatoes
11 1/2 ounces V-8® vegetable juice -- 1/ 11.5 oz can 1 can corn -- whole grains
1 can green beans - cut 1/2 teaspoon thyme - dried 1/4 teaspoon pepper
1 pound ground beef, extra lean
1 teaspoon garlic - chopped

Combine beef and garlic. Make meatballs and brown. Place meatballs and other ingredients in slow cooker and place over low heat for 6-8 hours.

Casserole of turkey with herbs and wild rice

6 slices of bacon, cut into 1/2-inch pcs.
1 lb turkey breast fillets, cut into 3/4-inch pcs.
1 med. onion, chopped (1/2 cup)
1 med. carrot, sliced (1/2 cup)
1 med. stem celery, sliced (1/2 cup)
2 cans (14 1/2oz) ready-to-serve chicken broth 1 can (10 3/4 oz) condensed cream of chicken soup 1/4 tsp dried marjoram leaves
1/8 tsp pepper
1 1/4 cups uncooked wild rice, rinsed and drained

Cook bacon in a 10-inch skillet over med heat. Stir in onion, carrot and celery. Cook, 2 min., stirring occasionally; Aspire. Beat a can of broth and soup in 3 1/2 qt. slow cooker, using a metal whisk, until smooth. Stir in remaining broth, marjoram and pepper. Stir in turkey mixture and wild rice. Cover and cook on HIGH for 30 min. Reduce heat to LOW. Cook for 6-7 hours. or until the rice is tender and the liquid is absorbed.

Per serving: cal 320, fat 8g, fat sat 3g, chol 60mg, turf 1140mg, carbohydrates 36g, fiber 3g, prot 29g
Made 6 servings

Herbed turkey breast

1 turkey breast, boneless and skinless (5 lbs)
2 T butter or margarine (light butter change)
1/4 t cream cheese flavoured with garden vegetables (probably could get light /FF) 1 T low sodium soy sauce
1 T fresh parsley - chopped
1/2 teaspoon basil - dried
1/2 tsp sage -- dried
1/2 tsp thyme --
dried
1/4 teaspoon ground black
pepper 1/4 teaspoon garlic
powder

Place turkey in sandstone. Mix remaining ingredients and brush turkey. Cover and cook over low heat for 10 to 12 hours or 5 to 6 hours. Makes 8 servings.

Nutritional information: 343 calories, 5 grams fat, 70 grams of protein, trace carbohydrates, 184 mg cholesterol, 244 mg sodium, trace fiber.

Hot crab dip
Makes 5 cups

1/2 cup skimmed
milk 1/3 cup salsa
3 pkgs. (8 oz each) light cream cheese, cubed
2 pkgs. (8 oz each) imitation of crab meat, flaked
1 cup minced green onions
1 can (4 oz) chopped green peppers

Combine milk and salsa. Transfer to a slow cooker covered with a non-stick spray. Stir in cream cheese, crab, onions and chillies. Cover and cook on LOW for 3 to 4 hours, stirring every 30 minutes.

Per (1/4 cup) serving: 80 cal, 385mg turf, 23mg chol,5g carbohydrates, 7g prot,3g fat

Fudge Crockpot Hot Cake

3 tbsp skimmed milk
1 can sugar-free cooking and serving chocolate pudding
1 box Super Moist chocolate fudge cake mix
1 1/3 ts where water is needed
1/2 tse apple 6 egg
whites

Spray a crockpot container with a non-greasy cooking spray. Whisk the skimmed milk with the dry pudding mixture in the slow cooker until dissolved. In a medium bowl, combine dry cake mixture, water, applesauce and egg whites with whisk for two minutes until mixed. Pour the cake mixture very gently over the pudding mixture. DON'T MIX IT UP! Cover and cook on HIGH for 2 1/2 hours. Serve hot Donne 15

Hot Texas chili soup

12 ounces red beans -- cooked and drained
6 ounces ground turkey -- cooked
3 cups canned simmered tomatoes -- low sodium
2 cups tomato sauce
1 1/2 cups chopped onions
1 cup canned green peppers, rinsed - drained and chopped 1
tablespoon and 2 teaspoons chili powder
1 1/2 teaspoons ground cumin
1 teaspoon paprika
1 teaspoon dried oregano
1/4 teaspoon hot pepper sauce

In 3 quarters slow cooker,combine all ingredients and 2 cups of water. Cover and cook over low heat for 4 hours or on High for 2 hours, until onions are tender. Ladle evenly in 6 soup bowls.
Each serving: (1 1/4 cups) provides: 2 proteins; 3 Vegetables. Per serving: 230 Calories, 15g. Protein; 5g. Fat; 35g. Carbohydrates; 104mg. Calcium; 569 mg sodium; 20mg. Cholesterol; 8g. Dietary fiber.

Hungarian Goulash

2 tablespoons vegetable oil
2 pounds beef stew, cut into inch pieces
1 large onion, sliced
14 1/2 ounces fat-free beef stock
6 ounces tomato paste
2 garlic cloves, finely chopped
1 tablespoon Worcestershire sauce
1 tablespoon paprika
1 teaspoon salt
1/4 teaspoon caraway seeds if desired 1/4
teaspoon pepper
1/4 cup cold water
3 tablespoons all-purpose flour
1 medium pepper, cut into strips
8 cups hot cooked noodles to serve

Heat oil in 10-inch skillet over medium-high heat. Cook beef in oil for about 10 minutes, stirring occasionally until golden; Aspire. Place beef and onion in a slow 3 1/2 to 6 litre stove. Combine broth, tomato paste, garlic, Worcestershire sauce, paprika, salt, caraway seeds and pepper; poivre; stir in beef mixture. Cover and cook over low heat for 8 to 10 hours until beef is tender. Mix water and flour; gradually stir in the beef mixture. Stir in pepper. Cover and cook over high heat for 30 minutes. Serve goulash over noodles.

Per serving: 417 calories; 13g fat; 38g protein; 37g carbohydrates; 3g dietary fibre; 108mg Cholesterol; 610mg sodium.

Italian beef and green pepper sandwiches

Makes 6 sandwiches

2 lbs fresh beef brisket
1 tbsp vegetable oil
1 can (10 1/2 oz) condensed beef stock
2 garlic cloves, finely chopped
1 tsp dried oregano leaves
1 tsp dried basil leaves 1/2
teaspoon salt
1/4 teaspoon pepper
1/4 tsp crushed red pepper
Two med. green peppers, cut into 1/4-
inch strips
12 slices of Italian or French crusty
bread, each about 1" thick

Cut off excess beef fat. Heat oil in 10-inch skillet over low heat. Cook beef in oil for about 10 min., turning occasionally, until both sides are brown. Place beef in a slow cookery of 3 1/2 to 6 qt. Mix remaining ingredients except peppers and bread; pour over the beef. Cover and cook on LOW 8-10 hours. or until the beef is tender. Remove beef from cutting board; thinly sliced. Cut the fat from beef juice in the stove. Stir the peppers into the juice. Cover and cook on HIGH for 15 minutes. Return the beef slices to the stove. Place 2 slices of bread on each plate. Pour the beef mixture over the bread.

Per sandwich: cal 300, fat 11g, sat fat 4g, chol 65mg, turf 720mg, carbohydrates 23g, fiber 2g

Italian Bow Tie Dinner

1/2 pound extra lean ground beef - brown and drained 1 medium
onion - chopped
1 clove garlic, chopped
8 ounces tomato sauce
14 1/2 Once canned tomatoes - stew
1 teaspoon dried oregano
1 teaspoon Italian seasoning salt
and pepper - to taste
8 Ounces Pasta - cooked and drained
10 ounces frozen spinach -- thawed and drained
1 cup mozzarella cheese, skimmed milk part - grated 1/2
cup fat-free Parmesan cheese

Place all ingredients, SAUF for cooked pasta, spinach and cheese) in a slow cooker. Cover and cook over low heat for 7 to 8 hours or until bubbly. Increase the slow cooker to high; stir in pasta, spinach and cheese. Cover and cook for 10 minutes or until hot and cheese is melted.

Per serving: 263 Calories); (kcal); 8g total fat; (26% calories from fat); 17g protein; 31g carbohydrates; 33mg Cholesterol; 424mg sodium

Italian pot roast

serves 8

1 round roast boneless egg (2 1/2-pond)
1 medium onion, sliced
1/4 teaspoon salt
1/4 teaspoon pepper
2 cans (8 ounces) salt-free tomato sauce
1 (0.7 ounces) Italian dressing mix

Slice the roast in half and place in a 3 1/2-quarter electric slow quartcooker. Add onion and remaining ingredients. Cover and cook over high heat for 5 hours or until roast is tender. Or, cover and cook at high setting 1 hour; reduce to low setting and cook for 7 hours. Slice the meat to serve.

Italian spaghetti sauce

2 pounds extra lean ground beef - or 'bulk Italian sausage 3 medium cut onions - (2-1/4 cups)
1 large green pepper -- chopped (1-1/2 cups) 6 garlic cloves -- finely chopped
29 ounces diced canned tomatoes -undated
29 ounces tomato sauce
12 ounces tomato paste
2 tablespoons dried basil leaves
1 tablespoon oregano leaves
1 tablespoon sugar -- or Splenda
1 teaspoon salt
1/2 teaspoon pepper
1/2 teaspoon crushed red pepper

Cook ground beef (or sausage), onions, pepper and garlic in a 12-inch skillet over medium heat for about 10 minutes, stirring occasionally, until meat is not pink; Aspire. Pour the meat mixture into a 5-litre Crock-Pot slow cooker. Stir in remaining ingredients. Cover and cook over low heat for 8 to 9 hours or until vegetables are tender.

24 servings (1/2 cup each) per serving: 128 Calories; 7g fat; 9g protein; 9g carbohydrates; 2g dietary fibre; 26mg Cholesterol; 485mg sodium.

Italian tortellini stew

1 onion, chopped
2 zucchini, sliced
32 oz chicken broth
28 oz crushed tomatoes
15 oz large Nordic beans
2 tbsp basil 1/4
teaspoon salt
1/4 teaspoon
pepper.
8 oz   tortellini filled with dry cheese

Combine all ingredients except tortellini in a slow cooker container. Cook over low heat for 6 hours. Turn heat to high and add tortellini. Cook 20 min. 8 servings

Italian Turkish rice dinner
Makes 4 servings

Three med. carrots, grated (2 cups)
Two med. celery stalks, sliced (1 cup)
1 small red pepper, chopped (1/2 cup) 1/2
teaspoon dried basil leaves
1/3 cup water
4 turkey legs (8-12 oz each), skin removed 1 tsp
salt
1/4 teaspoon pepper
1/2 cup uncooked regular long grain rice 1 tsp
dried oregano leaves
1/3 cup shredded Italian
mixture of six cheeses or mozzarella cheese (2 oz)

Combine carrots, celery, pepper, basil and water in 3 1/2-4 qt. Slow cooker. Sprinkle turkey with salt and pepper; place on the vegetable mixture.

Cover and cook on LOW for 6 to 7 hours. Remove turkey legs. Stir rice and oregano into vegetable mixture; put the turkey back in the slow cooker. Cover and cook on LOW around 1 hour or until rice is tender. Remove turkey legs. Stir cheese into rice mixture until melted. Serve with turkey.

Per serving: cal 370, fat 9g, fat sat 4g, chol 165mg, turf 810mg, carbohydrates 27g, fiber 2g, prot 47g

Italian dinner from Turkey
Makes 6 servings

2 turkey legs (1 lb), skin removed
1 (14.5 oz) can make diced tomatoes with Italian-style herbs, non-dramatic
2 tbsp tomato paste
2 garlic cloves, finely chopped
1 cup raw couscous
1 1/2 cups water
2 cups sliced zucchini

Place turkey legs in 3 1/2-4 qt. slow cooker. In a small bowl, combine tomatoes, tomato paste and garlic; mix well. Pour over turkey. Cover; cook on LOW for 6-8 hours. About 25 min. before serving, cook couscous in water as shown on pkg. Mix the zucchini in the tomato mixture. Cover; cook on HIGH for an additional 20 minutes or until zucchini are tender.

To serve, remove the bones from the turkey. Stir gently to break the turkey.

Par portion: cal 270 , gras 5 g , sat gras 2 g, chol 55 mg , glucides 31 g , fib 3 g , prot 24 g

Jambalaya

1 cup diced lean ham
2 onions, coarsely chopped
2 celery stalks, sliced
1/2 green pepper, seeded and chopped
1 (28 ounces) can whole tomatoes
1/4 cup tomato paste
3 garlic cloves, finely chopped
1 tablespoon chopped parsley 1/2
teaspoon dried thyme
2 whole cloves
1 tablespoon vegetable oil
1 cup long grain white rice
1 pound medium shrimp, peeled and deveined

In a slow cooker, combine ham, onions, celery, pepper, tomatoes, tomato paste, garlic, parsley, thyme, cloves, oil and rice. Cook on High 4-5 hours. Add shrimp and cook until prawns are pink, about 1 hour longer.

Per serving: 296 calories, 5 g total fat, 1 g saturated fat, 125 mg cholesterol, 513 mg sodium, 38 g total carbohydrates, 3 g dietary fiber, 24 g protein, 108 mg calcium.

Make-Ahead Fajitas

Makes 10 servings

Filling

1 1/2 lb beef flank steak, fat, cut into 32 strips 1 rag (1/2 cup)
onion, sliced
1 small (1/2 cup) green pepper, sliced
1 small (1/2 cup) red pepper, sliced
1 (1 oz) pkg. fajita seasoning mix
1 tbsp finely chopped fresh garlic

Tortillas

10 flour tortillas (8"), warmed

Pads

Cheddar cheese, grated, low-fat sour cream, Salsa, hot pepper sauce, Guacamole

Mix all the filling ingredients in a slow cooker. Cover; cook on LOW for 6-8 hours, or HIGH 3 - 4 hours. Drain the liquid. Cut or shred the meat, if desired. To serve, place meat mixture on hot tortillas. Garnish with desired garnishes. Per serving (without toppings):): cal 290, prot 20g, carbohydrates 31g, 2g fibre, 10g fat, 30mg chol, turf 530mg

Mom chicken stew

1 pound boneless chicken breasts, cut into bite-sized pieces 1 pound boneless chicken thighs, cut into bite-sized pieces 2 cups water
1 cup frozen whole onions
1 cup (1/2 inch) sliced celery
1 cup minced carrot
1 teaspoon paprika
1/2 teaspoon salt
1/2 teaspoon rubbed sage 1/2 teaspoon dried thyme 1/2 teaspoon black pepper
1 (14 1/4 ounces) can fat-free chicken broth
2 cups of mushrooms cut in half
1 (6 ounces) can stick tomato 1/4 cup water
3 tablespoons cornstarch
2 cups frozen green peas

Mix the first 14 ingredients in a large electric slow cooker. Cover with lid and cook over high heat for 4 hours or until carrot is tender. Whisk together water and cornstarch in a small bowl, whisking until mixed. Add cornstarch mixture and peas to slow cooker; stir well. Cover and cook over high heat, 30 minutes more. Yield: 8 servings (serving size: 1-1/2 cups).

CALORIES NUTRITIONAL INFORMATION 257; PROTEIN 30.8g; FAT 3.5g; CARB 25.1g; FIBER 2.8g; CHOL 78mg; IRON 3.2mg; SODIUM 359mg; CALC 83mg

Mexi Dip

16 ounces light cream cheese -- (2 8 oz pkg))
6 1/2 ounces canned ham flakes -- with liquid, crushed together 3 cups grated medium cheddar cheese
1/2 cup medium or hot Salsa
4 ounces canned chillies -- green, drained 1/2 teaspoon of chili powder -- 1/2 to 1 teaspoon.

Crush cream cheese with a fork in a bowl. extend into the bottom of 3-1/2 quarter slow cooker. Sprinkle ham evenly on top. Sprinkle with cheddar cheese. Combine salsa and green peppers. Pour over top. Sprinkle with chili powder. Cover. Cook over low heat for 2 to 2 and a half hours until hot enough. Do not stir. Yields 4 1/4

1 tablespoon servings

"When you dive with a chip or a sturdy spoon, you get different layers. Wrecks a lot of a diet. Serve with chips." Yield: "4 1/4 cups"

Per serving (excluding unknown items): 43 calories; 3g fat (70.3% calories from fat); 2g protein; 1 g carbohydrates; dietary fibre trace; 10mg cholesterol; 134mg sodium.

Mexican Green Chile

1 1/2 pounds lean top round,cut into 1-inch pieces
1 (16 ounces) jar tomatillo salsa (green salsa) (sweet is recommended) 1 (15 ounces) can Mexican-style simmered tomatoes
1 (15 ounces) fat-free beef stock
2 cans (4.5 ounces) chopped green peppers
1 cup chopped onion
2 teaspoons ground cumin
1 teaspoon freshly ground pepper
2 teaspoons bottled chopped garlic
2 teaspoons chili oil

Mix all ingredients in an electric slow cooker. Stir well. Cover. Cook over low heat for 8 hours.

Yield: 9 servings (1 cup) CAL: 156, FAT: 4 grams, FIBER: 1 gram, Protein: 19.3g; CARB: 8.7g; CHOL: 43MG; IRON: 2.1 mg; SODIUM: 675mg

Mom's homemade chicken soup

1 tablespoon vegetable oil
1 pound boneless skinless chicken breast halves -- cut into 1-inch 1 celery
medium-sized celery -- chopped (1/2 cup)
1 medium onion -- chopped (1/2 cup)
2 garlic cloves -- finely chopped
1 1/2 cups baby carrots -- quartered
1 tablespoon chicken broth granules
1 teaspoon dried thyme leaves
49 1/2 ounces ready-to-serve chicken broth 1 cup
frozen green peas
1 cup fine egg noodles

Heat oil in 10-inch skillet over medium-high heat. Cook chicken, stirring occasionally, until chicken is golden brown. Mix all ingredients except peas and noodles in a slow cooker of 3-1/2 to 4 quarter Crock-Pot. Cover and cook over low heat for 6 and a half to 7 hours or until vegetables are tender and chicken is no longer pink in the centre. Rinse frozen peas in cold water to separate; Aspire. Stir the peas and noodles into the soup. Cover and cook over high heat for about 15 minutes or until noodles are tender.

For 4 servings: 315 calories; 9g Fat; 34g Protein; 24g Carbohydrates; 4g Dietary Fibre; 75mg Cholesterol; 1868 mg Sodium.

Mustard onion chuck roast in foil

8 portions

2 tbsp dry mustard
1 1/2 teaspoons water
3-pound beef pot roast
2 medium onions, pieces of
one part and one cup of soy
sauce

Mix mustard and water to make a paste; let stand for 5 minutes. Place a piece of aluminum foil large enough to cover the meat in a shallow baking sheet; profonde; place the meat on foil. Sprinkle onion pieces over meat. Stir 1 tbsp soy sauce into mustard mixture, stirring until smooth; stir in remaining soy sauce. Pour the mixture evenly over the beef and onions. Fold foil over meat; seal securely. Roast at 325 for 3 hours.

Remove from the oven, cut the grain and serve with meatjuice..... Throw it at 3, it's ready to 6. IF DONE IN CROCKPOT, COOK 6 to 8 HOURS on LOW. Do not live the lid during cooking. I don't use aluminum foil in the slow cooker --- just put it all together.

No-Peek Chicken Casserole

2 pounds boneless skinless chicken breasts - cut into 1" pieces 1 wrap
dry onion soup mixture
1 can fat-free beef broth
1 can 98% fat-free cream of mushroom soup 4
ounces mushrooms - drained

Mix all ingredients in a slow cooker. Mix well. Cover and cook over low heat for 8 to 12 hours or high for 3 to 4 hours. Serve over noodles or rice. The recipe can be doubled. Per serving: 291 calories; 4g fat; 57g protein; 7g carbohydrates; 1g dietary fibre; 132mg Cholesterol; 1182mg sodium.

Poire Streusel

Makes 4 servings

1/3 cup crunchy walnut-shaped cereal
nuggets 3 tbsp all-purpose flour
3 tbsp light brown sugar
2 tbsp low-fat sweet margarine
1 tsp grated lemon zest 1/2
tsp ground ginger
4 Bartlett pears, peeled, cored and cut into 1/2-inch slices 3
tbsp fresh lemon juice
1/4 cup granulated sugar

In a small bowl, combine cereal, flour, brown sugar, margarine, lemon zest and ginger. Mix with a fork until crumbly; Set aside. In a 1 qt dish. a saucepan that fits into a slow cooker of 4 or 5 qt, mix the pears, lemon juice and granulated sugar. Sprinkle the mixture evenly on top. Place the pan in a slow cooker. Cover and cook over HIGH for 2 hours. or until pears are tender with a fork. Serve hot.

Per serving: cal 264, carb 60g, prot 2g, 4g fat, sat fat sat 0.5g, chol 0mg, turf 134mg
Also GREAT with apples instead of pears!!!!!

Beijing pork chops

6 pork chops, about 1" thick 1/4
c. brown sugar
1 tsp ground ginger
1/2 tsp soy sauce 1/4
tsp ketchup
1-2 cloves garlic, salt and
pepper purée, to taste

Cut excess fat from pork chops. Put the pork chops in the slow cooker. Combine brown sugar, ground ginger, soy sauce, ketchup, garlic, salt and pepper. Pour the mixture over the meat in a slow cooker. Cook, covered, over low heat for 4 to 6 hours, or until tender. Season with: salt and pepper (optional) Serve with: steamed white rice (we like jasmine rice) and/or Chinese noodles Notes: Made 6 servings. It works well with pork steaks too.

Hot Chicken Peles Sandwich
Makes 4-5 servings

1 lb boneless, skinless chicken breasts, cut into 2 x 1/2-inch strips
1 red pepper, cut into julienne strips
6 mushrooms, sliced
3/4 cup pineapple juice
2 tbsp. sauce teriyaki sauce
1 tbsp honey
1/2 teaspoon salt
1/8 to 1/4 teaspoon dried red pepper flakes
2 tsp Cornstarch
2 tbsp cold water
4-5 sesame bagels
1 small jicama, peeled and coarsely grated

Mix the first 9 ingredients in a 3 1/2 qt slow cooker. Cover and cook on LOW for about 4 hours. or until the chicken is tender. Turn the control to HIGH. In a small bowl, dissolve cornstarch in cold water. Stir in the contents of the slow cooker. Cover and cook for 15 to 20 minutes or until thickened. Meanwhile preheat the grill. Divide the bagels and place, cut the sides up, on a baking sheet. Grill under grill until lightly browned, about 5 min. Serve chicken mixture over bagels. Top with jucama..

Per serving: cal 373, carb 51g, prot 34g, 3g fat, sat sat 1g fat, chol 39mg, turf 856mg

Pepper steak in Crock

1 1/2 pounds flank steak - minced
1 large onion and slices
2 peppers -- all sliced color
2 tablespoons soy sauce
2 tablespoons sesame oil
1 tablespoon brown sugar
3 garlic cloves - sliced

Spray 3, 1/2 qt. crock with pam. Put everything in the slow cooker, mix well. Cook at low hours for 8 to 9 hours. Per serving: 269 calories; 16g fat; 23g protein; 7g carbohydrates; 1g dietary fibre; 58mg cholesterol; 424mg sodium

Pepsi and pork in the Crockpot
Donne 4 portions (3 oz)

1 (10 oz) can cream reduced fat mushroom soup
2 tbsp sodium-reduced soy sauce
1 (12 oz) can Pepsi Diet
4 pork chops (3 oz), well-prepared (or replace a roast pork)

Combine soup, soy sauce and Diet Pepsi together in the bottom of the Crockpot. Place chops in mixture and cook with high medication or high water content for 4-6 hours. The meat will be very tender.

Per serving: cal 213, fat 9g, prot 25g, carbohydrates 6g, 66mg, turf 434mg

Pineapple chicken

3 chicken breasts (split, peeled and boneless)
Pepper
Peppers
20 oz pineapple (drained, unsweetened sweets)
2 TB Mustard; Dijon soy
sauce
1 clove garlic; Chopped

Arrange chicken in slow cooker. Sprinkle with pepper and paprika. Combine soy sauce, pineapple and mustard; pour over the chicken. Add chopped garlic. Cover and cook on LOW 7 to 9 hours or on HIGH 3 to 4 hours. Makes 6 servings per serving: 210 calories; 4 g fat; 73 mg cholesterol; 153 mg sodium.

Pioneer beans

1 pound ground beef
1/4 pound sliced bacon - chopped 1
medium onion - chopped (1/2 cup)
1 15 ounces red beans -- rinsed and drained 1 15 ounces
buttered beans -- rinsed and drained
1 15 ounces pork and beans in tomato sauce 1 cup
catsup
1/2 cup packaged brown sugar -- (1/2-1)
1/4 cup molasses
1 tablespoon vinegar
1 tablespoon prepared mustard

In a large skillet, cook ground beef, ground bacon and onion until meat is no longer pink and onion is tender. Drain the fat. Stir in red beans and drained beans, pork and uns mossedbeans, catsup,brown sugar, molasses, vinegar and mustard. Transfer the mixture to a saucepan for 2 to 2 1/2 quarters. Cover and bake at 350oF for 30 minutes. Discover the pan; bake for another 30 minutes. Makes 12 servings. Crockery cook directions. Prepare the beans as directed, except transfer the meat and bean mixture to a 3 1/2 to 4-quarter electric dishwasher. Cover and cook over low heat for 5 to 6 hours, or over high heat for 2 and a half to 3 hours.

Calories... 256...Fat... 7g... Carbohydrates... 38g... Protein... 15g... Sodium... 684 mg... Fiber... Fourg.

Polynesian steak strips
Serves 6

2 lbs beef steak, cut through grain into thin slices 2 tbsp
Ketchup
1 tbsp oyster sauce 1/4
cup soy sauce 1/2 tsp
ground ginger 1/4 tsp
garlic powder
1 tsp granulated sugar
1/4 teaspoon liquid sauce
browning 1 tsp salt
1/4 teaspoon pepper

Place steak strips in 3 1/2 qt. slow cooker. Combine the remaining 10 ingredients in a small bowl. Pour on

Bands. Stir. Cover. Cook on LOW for 8 to 10 hours. or on HIGH for 4 to 5 hours.
Per serving: 263 cal,, 11.2 g fat, 1480 mg turf, 34 g prot,5 g carbohydrates

Pork meatballs with tomato sauce

Makes 24-26 meatballs

2 (8 oz) tomato sauce 1/4
teaspoon garlic powder
1/2 teaspoon ground
thyme 1/2 cup water
1 1/4 lbs lean ground beef 1/2
cup long grain rice
2 tbsp chopped onion
1/2 teaspoon salt
1/4 teaspoon ground black pepper

In a slow 1 1/2-qt cooker, combine tomato sauce, garlic powder, thyme and water. In a med bowl. Form in 24-26 balls the size of golf balls. Put the meatballs in the tomato mixture in a slow cooker. Cover and cook on LOW 7-8 hours. or until the rice is tender. Serve sauce over meatballs.

Per meatball: cal 80, carb 4g, prot 5g, 5g fat, sat fat 2g, chol 18mg, turf 118mg

Pork and black bean chili

1 LB roasted boneless boneless pork
1 (16 oz) thick, chunky salsa jar
2 (15 oz) of unsalted black bean cans, not
1 cup chopped yellow pepper 3/4 cup
chopped onion
1 teaspoon ground cumin
1 teaspoon of chili powder
1 teaspoon dried oregano 1/4
cup fat-free sour cream

Cut pork fat; cut into 1-inch pieces. Mix pork and the following 7 ingredients in a 4-quarter electric slow cooker; quarts; stir well. Cover with lid; cook over low heat for 8 hours or until pork is tender. Ladle chili in bowls; garnish with sour cream.

Yield: 4 servings (serving size: 2 cups chili and 1 tablespoon sour cream.
 Par portion : CAL 379; PRO 36,7g; FAT 9.4g (sam 2.8g); CARB 45.4g; FIB 14/2g; CHOL 62mg; IRON 6mg; SOD 405MG, CALC 136mg

Pork chop dinner
Makes 6 servings

6 pork loin chops (3/4" thick)
1 tbsp vegetable oil
1 large onion, sliced
1 med. green pepper, chopped
1 can (4 oz) mushroom stalk and pcs., drained
1 can (8 oz) tomato sauce
1 tbsp brown sugar
2 tsp Worcestershire sauce
1 1/2 teaspoons cider
vinegar 1/2 teaspoon salt
Hot cooked rice (optional)

In a frying pan, brown pork chops on both sides in oil; Aspire. Place chops in a slow cooker. Add onion, green pepper and mushrooms. In a bowl, combine tomato sauce, brown sugar, Worcestershire sauce, vinegar and salt. Pour over meat and vegetables. Cover and cook low in 4-5 hours. or until the meat is tender. Serve with rice if desired.

Per serving without rice: 199 cal, 8g fat, 2g sat fat, sat59mg chol,507mg turf,

Pork chops with Jalapeno-Pecan cornbread stuffing
Makes 6 servings

6 boneless pork loin chops, 1 inch thick (1 1/2 lbs) 3/4
cup chopped onion
3/4 cup chopped celery
1/2 cup pecans, coarsely chopped
1/2 med. jalapeno pepper, seeded and chopped 1 tsp
rubbed sage
1/2 tsp dried rosemary leaves 1/8
teaspoon black pepper
4 cups unskilled cornbread stuffing mixture
1 1/4 cups reduced sodium chicken stock
1 egg, lightly beaten

Cut off excess pork fat and discard. Spray a large frying pan with a non-stick spray; heat over med heat. Add pork; cook onion, celery, pecans, jalapeno pepper, sage, rosemary and black pepper in skillet. Bake for 5 minutes or until tender. Book. Mix the stuffing mixture with the cornbread, the vegetable mixture and the broth in the med bowl. Stir in egg. Pour the stuffing mixture into the slow cooker. Arrange the pork on top. Cover and cook on LOW for about 5 hours. or until the pork is tender and barley pink in the centres.

Tip: If you prefer a moist dressing, increase chicken broth to 1 1/2 cups. Per serving: cal 272, fat 14g, prot 17g, carbohydrates 19g, chol 75mg, turf 380mg, fiber 1g

Pork chops and potatoes with mustard sauce

6 4-ounce pork loin chops - adorned
1 10 3/4 ounces can Campbell's 98% Fat Free Cream of Mushroom Soup 1/4 cup
low sodium chicken broth
1/4 cup Dijon mustard 1/2
teaspoon dried thyme
1 clove garlic -- chopped, or 1/4 teaspoon garlic
powder 1/4 teaspoon black pepper
6 medium potatoes -- thinly sliced
1 onion - sliced

In the pan, brown pork chops in 2 tablespoons of oil, if desired. In any size Crockpot Slow Cooker, combine soup, chicken broth, mustard, thyme, garlic and pepper. Stir in potatoes and onion to coat. Place the golden pork chops on top of the potato mixture. Cover and cook on LOW for 8 to 10 hours or on HIGH 4 to 5 hours.

Per serving: 240 calories); (kcal); 6g total fat; 18g protein; 28g carbohydrates; 38mg cholesterol; 565 mg sodium

Pizza pot

8 ounces lean ground beef or turkey 1/2 cup
chopped onion
1/2 cup chopped green pepper
1/2 cup (a 2.5-ounce jar) sliced mushrooms, drained
1 3/4 cup (a 15-ounce can) Hunt 'lt tomato sauce; -I used Hunt's pizza sauce 1 teaspoon
Italian seasoning
1 teaspoon Spenda pourable
3 cups cooked noodles, rinsed and drained
1/4 cup grated Kraft Reduced Fat Cheddar Cheese 1/4 cup
reduced-fat Kraft shredded Mozzarella cheese

In a large frying pan, sprinkled with cooking spray flavoured with olive oil, brown meat, onion and green pepper. Stir in mushrooms, tomato sauce, Italian seasoning and Splenda. Pour the mixture into a spray slow cooker with a butter-flavoured cooking spray. Spread noodles over meat mixture. Sprinkle with Parmesan cheese. Spread cheddar and mozzarella cheeses evenly on top.
Cover and cook on LOW for 6-8 hours/ Mix well before serving
Makes 6 (1 cup) 305 calories, 9 fat gm,, 21 gm proteins, , 35 gm carbohydrates, , 866 mg sodium, 209 gm Calcium, 4 gm fiber

Roast

4 large potatoes -- cut into pieces
4 large carrots -- cut into pieces
2 large onions -- cut into pieces
2 cups rutabaga - cut into pieces
3 pounds boneless beef broth (or other) - cut 1/2 cup boiling
water
1 teaspoon beef broth granules 1/2
teaspoon liquid sauce browning

Place potato, carrot, rutabaga and onion in a slow 5 litre stove. Place the roast on top. Combine the remaining 3 ingredients in a small bowl. Stir. Pour over top. Cover. Cook on LOW for 10 to 12 hours or on HIGH for 5 to 6 hours. Serves 8 to 10. (I sometimes use a packet of onion soup mixture instead of browner liquid sauce and beef broth granules, and use 3/4 cups of boiling water. Per serving: 273 calories; 10g fat; 33g protein; 16g carbohydrates; 3g dietary fibre; 116mg cholesterol;141mg sodium.

Potato and leek chowder

3 medium potatoes - peeled and diced
11 ounces canned corn, 1/2 cup
chopped celery
1 leek soup, packet
4 cups water
1 cup non-greasy dry milk powder
1/2 cup grated Swiss cheese

In slow cooker, combine potatoes, corn, celery, dry leek soup mixture and water. Cover and cook on LOW for 5 to 6 hours or until potatoes and celery are tender. Just before serving, gradually add the dry milk powder to the hot soup; whisk gently until well blended. Ladle in individual soup bowls; individuels; sprinkle with cheese, if desired.

Chowder de pomme de terre et de mushrooms

1/2 cup onion -- chopped
1/4 cup reduced-calorie margarine 2
tablespoons flour
1 teaspoon salt
1/2 teaspoon black pepper 2
cups water
8 ounces sliced mushrooms, drained -- fresh can be used 1 cup
celery -- chopped
2 cups potatoes - peeled and diced
1 cup carrots -- chopped
2 cups skim milk
1/4 cup fat-free Parmesan cheese -- grated

In a frying pan, brown onion and celery in one-and-a-half cup margarine until onion is translucent. Remove from heat. Add flour, salt and pepper; Stir. Place in a pot of slow cooker. Add water, then stir in potatoes, mushrooms and carrots. Cover and cook at low 6-8 hours (or long for 3-4 hours). If on the bottom, turn high after cooking time. Add milk and Parmesan cheese and cook for another 30 minutes. Serve.
Per serving: 150 calories; 4g fat; 7g Prot;23g Carb;3g Fibre; 5mg Cholesterol; 718mg Sodium.

Red beans and rice
Makes 8 servings

1 lb dried beans (2 cups), sorted and rinsed 1 large green
pepper, chopped (1 1/2 cups)
1 large onion, chopped (1 cup)
2 garlic cloves, finely chopped
7 cups water
1 1/2 teaspoons
salt 1/4 teaspoon
pepper
2 cups raw instant rice Red
pepper sauce

Mix all ingredients except rice and pepper sauce in a slow cookery of 3 1/2 to 6 qt. Cover and cook over HIGH for 4-5 hours. or until the beans are tender. Stir in rice. Cover and cook on HIGH for 15 to 20 minutes or until rice is tender. Serve with pepper sauce.

Per serving: cal 250, fat 1g, sat fat 0g, chol 0mg, turf 460mg, carbohydrates 57g, fib 10g, prot 14g

Fried beans

2 lbs dried pinto beans
2-3 onions
1 tbsp salted water
3-4 slices of bacon (optional)
chopped peppers (optional)

Sort the beans to remove any non-bean objects such as rocks. Pour the beans into a large saucepan and add water to cover the beans at a depth of 2-3 inches. Soak beans for at least eight hours or bring water to a boil and simmer for an hour and a half. At the end of this time, stir the beans (to float the sediments) and pour in the water. Rinse beans once or twice as much to make sure they are clean. Fill the pan with enough water for the beans to be covered after they are lined in bulk. Chop the onions and peppers and bacon into pieces. [The heat and flavour of the pepper will soften during the cooking process; If you want heat, then either save them for later or use more than you think you need.] Add all the ingredients except the salt to the pan. Bring water to a boil and reduce to a boil. Cover and cook for 3 to 4 hours or until beans are very tender and tender, stirring occasionally and adding water as needed to keep beans covered. Add salt to about 2.5 hours.

Rustic vegetable soup

16 elevens spicy willow -- (1 pot)
10 ounces frozen mixed vegetables -- thawed (1 pkg.) 10
ounces frozen green beans -- cut, thawed, (1 pkg.) 10 ounces
fat-free beef stock
2 medium cooking potatoes -- cut into 1/2-inch pieces
1 medium green pepper -- chopped 1/2
teaspoon sugar
1/4 cup parsley

Mix all ingredients except parsley in slow cooker. Cover and cool on LOW for 8 hours or on HIGH for 4 hours. Stir the parsley; serve.
Per serving: 98 calories; Grease; 5g Prot;21g Carb;3g Dietary Fiber;0mg Chol;572mg Sod NOTES: I added 2 cans of fat-free condensed beef broth, 2 cans of water, 2 bay leaves, 1 tsp basil leaves

Chicken salsa

4 portions.

1 lb boneless, skinless chicken breast
1 bo salsa
2 tbsp flour

Place chicken and salsa in a slow cooker that ends with salsa. Cook low for 10-12 hours. When ready to serve, turn the slow cooker high and stir in 2 tablespoons of flour. Cook until thickened. I serve it with rice. If you have leftovers, shred the chicken and put it in a low-fat flour tortilla with fat-free sour cream and fat-free grated cheese.

Sausage pasta stew

1 lb of Italian turkey Sausage links, case removed
4 cups water
1 jar (26oz) meatless spaghetti sauce
1 can (16oz) red beans, rinsed and drained
1 medium yellow summer squash, halved lengthwise and cut into 1-inch 2 medium carrots, cut into half-inch slices
1 medium sweet red or green pepper, diced 1/3 cup chopped onion
1 1/2 cups raw spiral pasta
1 cup frozen peas
1 tsp sugar 1/2 teaspoon salt
1/4 teaspoon pepper.

In a non-stick skillet, cook sausages over medium heat until no longer pink; drain and place in a 5qt slow cooker. Add water, spaghetti sauce, beans, summer squash, carrots, red pepper and onion; mix well. Cover and cook over low heat for 7 to 9 hours or until vegetables are tender.

Stir in pasta, peas, sugar, salt and pepper; mix well. Cover and cook over high heat for 15 to 20 minutes or until pasta is tender. For portions: 8 (1 1/3 cups) Calories 276; Fat 6g; Fibre 6g

Dinner sausage and sauerkraut

Makes 4 servings

6 small red potatoes, unpeeled, in quarters
8 fresh carrots, cut into 1/4-inch slices
1 med. onion, cut into thin wedges
1 Tbs. brown sugar
1 tbsp spicy brown mustard
1 tsp caraway seeds
1 (15oz) can sauerkraut
1 lB fully cooked kielbasa turkey, cut into 1-inch slices

In a 3 1/2-4 qtslowcooker, combine potatoes, carrots and onion. In a medium bowl, mix brown sugar, mustard and caraway seeds - mixwell. Stir in sauerkraut and kielbasa. Pour this mixture over the vegetables in a cookery. Cover, cook on LOW for at least 8 hours. Per serving: 360 cal,7g fat, 7g fibre

Tasty beef fajitas
Makes 12 servings

1 beef rib steak (2 lbs) thinly sliced
1 cup tomato juice
2 garlic cloves, finely chopped
1 tbsp chopped fresh coriander or parsley 1
tsp chili powder
1 tsp ground cumin
1/2 teaspoon salt
1/2 tsp ground coriander 1
med. onion, sliced
1 med. green pepper, julienne
1 med. jalapeno, cut into thin strips
12 flour tortillas (7")
Sour cream, guacamole, salsa or grated cheddar cheese, optional

Put the beef in a slow cooker. Mix the following 7 ingredients; pour over the beef. Cover and cook on LOW for 6 to 7 hours. Add onions, pepper and jalapeno. Cover and cook for 1 hour longer or until meat and vegetables are tender. Using a slotted spoon, place about 1/2 cup of meat vegetable mixture on each tortilla. Add the desired toppings. Roll it up.

Per serving (without toppings):): 225 cal 7g fat, 3g sat fat, sat39mg chol, 254mg turf, 19g carbohydrates, 2g fiber, 20g prot

Roast savorrie pot
8 serv.

3-3 1/2 pound roasted chuck boneless beef
1 tbsp vegetable oil
8 small red potatoes, halved
3 cups carrots, cut by baby
1 large onion, coarsely chopped (1 cup)
1 jar (5 ounces) prepared horseradish
1 tsp salt
1/2 teaspoon
pepper 1 cup
water

Cut the fat from the roast. Heat oil in skillet over medium-high heat. Cook beef in oil for about 10 minutes, turning occasionally, until golden on all sides. Place potatoes, carrots and onion in a 4 to 6 litre slow cooker. Place beef on top of vegetables. Combine horseradish, salt and pepper; spread evenly over the beef. Pour water over beef and vegetables. Cover and cook over low heat for 8 to 10 hours or until beef and vegetables are tender. Special Notes This is my favorite pot roast.... horseradish gives it a good taste, but not horseradish -Calories:315; Fat: 13g; Fibre: 4g

Sirloin Tip Casserole

2 1/2 lbs of sirloin tips
1 can campbell's mixture of golden mushroom soup
1 pkg. Onion Soup Mix
Small whole potatoes

In the whole crook pot mixture 2 1/2 lbs sirloin tips, 1 can Campbell's blend of golden mushroom soup, and 1 pkg. Onion Soup Mix Peel as many small whole potatoes as you desire and place on top of the meat mixture - turning them once to cover them with the soup mixture so they brown well. Serve with your favourite vegetable and crusty bread. That's a lot of sauce - believe it or not.

Beef slowly cooked Burgundy

1/3 cup flour All-purpose 1
teaspoon salt
1/4 teaspoon pepper
2 lbs beef stew cubed
1 1/2 cups fresh carrots, halved in a cross-cutting direction
1 (10 oz) fresh pearl onions, peeled
1 (8 oz) pkg. fresh whole mushrooms
1 clove garlic, finely chopped
1 bay leaf
1 (10 1/2 oz) can condensed consumed beef
1 1/2 cups water
Fresh oregano, if desired

In a slow 3 1/2- or 4-quarter cooker, combine flour, salt, pepper and beef; mix well. Add all remaining ingredients; mix well. Cover; cook in a LOW setting for 10 to 12 hours or until carrots and beef are tender. Garnish with oregano.

NUTRITION INFORMATION PER SERVING: Calories 340 Fat10 g Dietary Fiber 3g 5 portions
de 1 2/3 tasse

Simmer slowly cooked chicken and sausage stew

1-1/2 cups serving 4 (1 1/2 cups of servings)
1/2 lb Kielbasa sausage, cut into 1/4-inch slices
2 boneless, skinless chicken breast halves, cut into bite-sized strips (I use 1 LB) 1/2 cup
minced carrot
1 small onion, thinly sliced
1 (16oz) baked beans, not
2 tbsp brown sugar
1 tsp dry mustard
1/2 cup ketchup
1 tbsp vinegar
2 cups thawed frozen cut green beans

In 3 1/2 to 4 quarters of Crock Pot, combine all ingredients except green beans. Cover, cook at low setting for 6 to 8 hours or until chicken is no longer pink. Ten minutes before serving, stir in the green beans. Increase heat to high; cover and cook for another 10 minutes or until green beans are tender.

Calories - 460 Fat 18 gr Fiber 8 gr Protein 28 gr

Slow-cooked chicken cacciatore

4 chicken thighs -- skin removed if desired
4 chicken thighs -- skin removed if desired
I (l5-oz.) Can Chunky sauce tomate de style italien
1 4.5 Oz Jar Green Giant' Whole Mushrooms - drained 1
teaspoon dried oregano leaves
1 small onion - sliced
1 small green pepper -- cut into 1-inch pieces 2 garlic
cloves - finely chopped
1/4 cup water
2 tablespoons Pillsbury Best' All Purpose or Unbleached Flour

In a 4qt.slow stove, combine all ingredients except water and flour; mix gently. Cover; cook at low setting for 6 to 8 hours. Using a slotted spoon, remove chicken and vegetables from slow cooker; place in a serving bowl. Cover to keep warm.

In a small bowl, combine water and flour: mix well. Stir the liquid into a slow cooker. Increase heat to high; cover and cook for an additional 5 to 10 minutes or until thickened. Stir well; mixture of spoons on chicken If desired, serve with hot cooked pasta.
Per serving (NOTES: 340 cal., 17 g. fat, 105 mg chole., 690 mg turf, 14 g. catbs.,3 g. fiber, 8 g. sugar

Slow-cooked garlic chicken

Serves 4

4 skinned chicken breast halves
1 teaspoon salt
2 teaspoons paprika
2 teaspoons lemon pepper
1 large onion, sliced
10 garlic cloves (about 1 medium), unpeeled

Combine salt, pepper and paprika. Rub on the chicken breast meat side. Place onion in slow cooker. Place the chicken breast side on top of the onion. Place garlic on chicken. Cover and cook over low heat in a slow cooker for about 6 hours or until juice is clear.

Roast pork with honey-Dijon cooked slowly

Makes 8 servings

1/2 cup chopped onion
2 apples, peeled and sliced
1 tbsp honey
1 tsp Dijon mustard
1/2 teaspoon coriander seeds,
crushed 1/4 teaspoon salt
1 (2 to 2 1/2 lbs) boneless pork roast rolled 1
tsp Cornstarch
2 tbsp water

In 4 to 6 qt. slow cooker,mix onion and apples. In a small bowl, combine honey, mustard, coriander and salt; mix well. Spread on all sides of the roast pork; place the roast on the onions and apples. Cover; cook on LOW for 7-8 hours. Remove roast from slow cooker; place on the serving tray. Cover with aluminum foil.

In a small saucepan, mix cornstarch and water, mix well. Add apple mixture and slow cooker juices; mix well. Cook over the med. heat until the mixture boils, stirring occasionally. Slice the roast. Serve with sauce.
Per serving: cal 250, 10g fat, 4g sat fat, sat chol 85mg, turf 180mg, carbohydrates 9g, fib 1g, prot 31g

Sweet and sour pork cooked slowly

1 1/2 pounds pork loins, lean, boneless - cubed
8 ounces canned pineapple pieces in juice - non-dedrain (unsweetened juice) 1 medium
red pepper - cut into squares or green pepper
3 tablespoons brown sugar 1/2
teaspoon ginger
1/4 cup vinegar
3 tablespoons soy sauce
3 tablespoons water
2 tablespoons cornstarch
2 cups cooked rice

In a slow cooker of 3-1/2 to 4 liters, combine pork, pineapple, pepper, brown sugar, ginger, vinegar and soy sauce. Mix well. Cover; cook on the LOW setting for 6 to 8 hours. About 5 minutes before serving, in a small bowl, mix 3 tablespoons of water and cornstarch; maïs; mix well. Stir pork mixture into a slow cooker. Cover; cook over high heat for an additional 5 minutes or until thickened. Serve pork mixture over rice. Makes 4 servings

Prepare the rice 25 minutes before serving.

Per serving: 410 calories; 8g fat; 34g protein; 49g carbohydrates; 2g dietary fibre; 77mg Cholesterol; 841mg sodium.

Turkey dinner simmered

6 small red potatoes -- unpeeled, quartered (about 2 1/2 inches in diameter) 2 cups
sliced carrots
1 1/2 pounds dark turkey meat, skinless -- (turkey legs) 1/4 cup
all-purpose flour
2 tablespoons onion soup mixture - dry
1/3 cup chicken broth
1 can condensed cream reduced mushroom soup fat

Place potatoes and carrots in 3-1/2 or 4-quarter Crock-Pot® Slow Cooker. Place turkey legs on vegetables. In a medium bowl, combine flour and remaining ingredients; mix well. Pour well. Pour over turkey. Cover; cover in high setting for 30 minutes.

Reduce the setting to low; cook for at least 7 hours or until turkey if tender fork. Using a slotted spoon, remove turkey and vegetables from slow cooker; place on the serving tray. Mix sauce until smooth; pour over turkey and vegetables.

Per serving: 424 calories; 10g fat;; 40g protein; 42g Carbohydrates; 5g dietary fibre; 118mg cholesterol; 1387mg sodium.

NOTES: For best results: Fill a slow cooker from half to three quarters full. Use lean meats, cut off any extra fat, and skinless poultry to reduce fat in slow-cooked meals. Thaw frozen ingredients in your microwave before adding to slow cooker, so they cook well. Remove the lid only to stir food or check for certainty. Lifting the lid releases heat, and the dish may require extra cooking time.

Roasted cooker Turkey and vegetables
Makes 4 servings

1 cup barbecue sauce
1/2 cup hot water
2 turkey legs (2 lbs), skin removed, halved, unpeeled,
cut into 8 pcs. Each 6 m2 of carrots, cut into 2 1/2x
1/2 inch sticks

In the med bowl. bien mix well. Place turkey, potatoes and carrots in a slow 3 1/2 to 4 qt stove. Pour the sauce mixture over the top. Cover; cook on LOW for at least 9 hours. Remove turkey and vegetables with a slotted spoon; place on the serving tray. Serve with cooking juices over turkey and vegetables.

Par portion: cal 380 , gras 9 g , sat gras 3 , chol 85 mg , sod 630 mg , carb 42 g , fib 6 g

Slow Cooker BBQ Short Ribs
Serves 6

2 tbsp cooking oil
3 lbs short beef ribs
1 cup BBQ sauce
2 c. Molasses
2 tbsp white vinegar
1 1/2 teaspoons
salt 1/2 teaspoon
pepper 1 tbsp soy
sauce
1/2 cup chopped onion

Heat the cooking oil in a frying pan. Add ribs. Brown on all sides. Aspire. Place ribs in 5 qt. slow cooker. Mix the following 6 ingredients in a bowl. Stir in onion. Pour over short ribs. Cook on LOW for 8 to 10 hours. or on HIGH for 4 to 5 hours. Per serving: 310cal, 15.9 g fat, 1415 mg turf, 27 g prot,13 g carbohydrates

Short slow cooker beef ribs
Serves 8

4 lbs short beef ribs, sprinkled with salt
Sprinkle with pepper
2 qniles, sliced or chopped
2 tsp ground beef stock 1/2
teaspoon liquid sauce browning
1 1/2 cups hot water

Sprinkle short ribs with salt and pepper. Place the onion in the bottom of the 5 qt slow cooker. Arrange the ribs on top. Stir broth powder and browning of sauce into hot water. Pour over the ribs. Cover. Cook on LOW for 7 to 9 hours. or on HIGH for 3 1/2-4 1/2 hours.

Per serving: 215cal, 11.9g fat, 203 mg turf, 23g prot,3g carbohydrates

Simmer Brunswick Stew
Makes 10 servings

1 1/2 lbs skinless, boneless chicken breasts, cut into 1 pcs. 3 m.
potatoes, cut into 1/2-inch pcs.
1 med. carrot, chopped (1/2 cup)
1 can (28 oz) crushed tomatoes, not
1 can (15 to 16 oz) lima beans, rinsed and drained 1 can
(14 3/4 oz) creamed corn
1 tbsp Worcestershire sauce
3/4 tsp salt
1/2 tsp dried marjoram leaves
8 slices bacon, cooked and crumbled 1/4
teaspoon red pepper sauce

Combine all ingredients except bacon and red pepper sauce in a slow cookery 3 1/2 to 6 qt. Cover and cook on LOW 8-10 hours (orHIGH 3-4 hours.) or until potatoes are tender. Stir in bacon and pepper sauce. Per serving: cal 250, fat 6 g, sat fat 2 g, cho 50 mg, sod 630 mg, carb 31 g, fib 6g, prot 24g

Jambalaya slow cooker
Serves 8

1 cup chopped onion
1 cup green pepper, chopped
1 cup chopped celery
3 garlic cloves, finely chopped
1 (28 oz) can de-control diced   tomatoes
2 cups fully cooked smoked sausage, copped 1/2
teaspoon parsley flakes
1/2 teaspoon salt
1/4 teaspoon dried thyme
leaves 1/4 teaspoon red pepper
sauce
3/4 lb uncooked peeled med, thawed if frozen 4 cups hot cooked rice

Mix all ingredients except shrimp and rice in 3 1/2-6 qt. slow cooker. Cover and cook low in 7-8 hours. or until the vegetables are tender. Stir in shrimp. Cover and cook over low heat for about 30 minutes or until prawns are pink and firm. Serve with rice.

Per serving: cal 245, 10g fat, 4g sat fat, sat   60mg chol, 700mg turf, 30g carbohydrates, 2g fib,   prot 11g

Slow cooker chicken merlot

serves 6

3 cups fresh mushrooms, sliced
1 onion, chopped
2 garlic cloves, finely chopped
3 lbs skinless chicken pieces, breasts, thighs, drumsticks, rinsed 3/4 cup
chicken stock
6 ounces tomato paste
1/4 cup dry red wine, such as merlot, or chicken broth 2 Tbs.
quick cooking tapioca
2 tsp sugar
1-1/2 tsp dried basil, crushed, or 2 tbs. fresh, cut 2 cups
cooked noodles
2 tbsp grated Parmesan cheese

Mix the first 3 ingredients and salt and pepper to taste in a slow cookery of 3-1/2 to 5 liters. Arrange chicken pieces over vegetables. Combine the broth according to 4 ingredients and the salt and pepper to taste in a bowl. Add dried basil if using. Pour over chicken. Cover and cook at low hours for 7 to 8 hours or over high heat for about 4 hours. Stir in fresh basil now if using. Serve noodles, sprinkled with Parmesan cheese. Because this recipe is for a particular size pan, it adjusts the number of servings only in multiples of 6.

Per serving: 381 calories, fat 4.1g, 10% fat calories, 133mg cholesterol, protein 57.6g, carbohydrates 24.9g, fibre 2.9g, sugar 4.5g, sodium 499mg, diet

Soupe Chili Slow-Cooker

1 tablespoon oil
1 1/2 pounds boneless round beef steak -- cut into 1/2-inch cubes 1
1/2 cups water
1 cup onions -- chopped
1 cup pepper -- chopped 1/2
teaspoon salt
1/2 teaspoon pepper
1/2 teaspoon cayenne pepper 1/4
teaspoon garlic powder
29 ounces peeled tomatoes, diced
15 1/2 ounces tomato sauce
1 cup carrots -- chopped
31 ounces dark red beans -- drained

Once the beef is golden in a frying pan, pour into the slow cooker with the vegetables and spices. Cook for 4 to 5 hours at low setting until finished.

Per serving: 383 calories; 13g fat; 28g protein; 41g carbohydrates; 10g dietary fibre; 50mg cholesterol; 545mg sodium.

Slow Cooker Double Onion Beef Sandwiches

Makes 8 sandwiches

3 large garlic cloves, finely chopped
1 tbsp Worcestershire sauce 1/2
teaspoon coarsely ground pepper
3 lbs fresh beef breast (no corned beef)
1 med. onion, thinly sliced
1 pkg. (1.3 oz) onion soup mixture
1/2 cup water
8 individual French rolls or crusty rolls

Combine garlic, Worcestershire sauce and pepper; rub on both sides of the beef. Cut the beef in half or three to fit the slow cooker. Place the sliced onion in the bottom of 3/2-6 qt. slow cooker. Garnish with pieces of beef; sprinkle with soup mixture (dry). Add water. Cover and cook low in 8-10 hours. or until the beef is tender. Remove beef; cut through the grain into these slices. Cut the fat from the juice in the slow cooker. Cut the buns horizontally in half. Fill the bread with beef. Drizzle with juice.

Per serving: cal 410, fat 14g, fat sat 5g, chol 95mg, turf 680mg, carb 31g, fiber 3g, prot 42g

Enchiladas mijoteuses

1 lb ground beef (ground turkey)
1 onion, chopped
1/2 tst chopped green pepper
1 can of red beans, rinsed and drained
1 can diced tomatoes w/ Green peppers,, not-- undraded
1 small can of tomato sauce
1 pkg. taco seasoning, dry
1/3 cup water
1/2 teaspoon
salt 1/4
teaspoon pepper
1 cup grated-fat reduced cheese (I used fat-free) 6 flour
tortillas

In skillet, cook beef, onion and green pepper until golden. Aspire. In a bowl, add all other ingredients except tortillas and stir. In the layer of crockpot 3/4 beef mixture, then tortilla. Repeat the layers with the 6 tortillas. Cover and cook over low heat for 5 to 7 hours. 6 servings

Tarte Tamale Slow Cooker Fiesta

3/4 cup yellow cornmeal 1
cup beef stock
1 lb extra-lean ground beef
1 tsp chili powder 1/2
tsp ground cumin
1 jar (14 to 16 oz) thick and thick salsa 1 (16 oz)
can whole grain corn, drained 1/4 cup sliced
ripe olives
2 oz low-fat cheddar cheese, grated (1/2 cup)

In a large bowl, combine cornmeal and broth; let stand for 5 minutes. Stir in beef, chili powder, cumin, salsa, corn and olives. Pour into a 3 1/2 qt slow cooker. Cover and cook on LOW 5 to 7 hours. or until it is settled. Sprinkle cheese on top; cover and cook for another 5 minutes or until cheese melts.

Per serving: cal 350, carb 34g, prot 21g, fat 16g, sat fat 0g, chol 57mg, turf 935mg

Slow Cooker Georgia-Style Barbecued Turkey Sandwich
Makes 12 sandwiches

4 turkey legs (2 1/2 to 3 lbs), skin removed 1/2 cup
of solidly packaged brown sugar
1/4 cup prepared mustard 2
tbsp Ketchup
2 tbsp cider vinegar
2 tbsp Louisiana-style hot pepper sauce
1 tsp salt
1 tsp coarsely ground black pepper
1 tsp crushed red pepper flakes
2 tsp liquid smoke
12 sandwich buns, split
1/2 pint (1 cup) creamy cabbage salad (deli)

Spray 4-6 qt. slow cooker with a non-stick spray. Place turkey in a slow cooker. In a small bowl, combine all remaining ingredients except buns and coleslaw; mix well. Pour over turkey, turning turkey as needed to coat. Cover; cook on LOW for 8-10 hours. Remove turkey from slow cooker; place on a large plate. Remove meat from bones; discard the bones. Tear the turkey with 2 forks. Return turkey to broth; mix well. To serve, using a slotted spoon, place about 1/3 cup of turkey mixture on the bottom half of each loaf. Garnish each with rounded tablespoons. Cover with top halves of buns.

Per serving: cal 260, fat 6g, fat sat 2g, chol 45mg, turf 560mg, fib 2g, prot 18g

Hot German slow cooker potato salad
Makes 6 servings

5 m. potatoes (about 1 3/4 lbs), cut into 1/4-inch slices 1
large onion, chopped
1/3 cup water
1/3 cup cider vinegar 2
tbsp all-purpose flour 2
tbsp. Sugar
1 tsp salt
1/2 tsp celery seeds
1/4 teaspoon pepper
4 slices crispy cooked bacon, crumbled

Mix potatoes and onion in 3 1/2-6 qt. slow cooker. Mix remaining ingredients except bacon; pour into the stove. Cover and cook on LOW 8-10 hours. or until the potatoes are tender. Stir in bacon.

Par portion: cal 160 , gras 2 g , sat gras 1 g , cho 5 mg , sod 470 mg , carb 35 g , fib 3 g , prot 4 g

Spaghetti Slow-Marinara Sauce
Makes 12 servings

2 cans (28 oz each) italian herb crushed tomatoes 1 can (6 oz)
tomato paste
1 large onion, chopped (1 cup)
8 garlic cloves, finely chopped
1 tbsp olive oil or vegetable oil
2 tsp sugar
1 tsp dried oregano leaves
1 tsp salt
1 tsp pepper
12 cups hot cooked spaghetti to serve grated
Parmesan cheese, if desired

Mix all ingredients except spaghetti and cheese in a slow cookery 3 1/2 to 6 qt. Cover and cook on LOW 8 to 10 hours. (orou HIGH 4 to 5 hours.) Serve over spaghetti. Sprinkle with cheese.

Par portion: cal 255 , gras 2 g , sat gras 0 g , cho 0 mg , sod 670 mg , carb 54 g , fib 4 g , prot 9 g

Slow cooker meatloaf
(Gele well)

24 ounces ground turkey or extra lean beef
1 cup finely chopped onion
4 slices of white bread with reduced calorie content, torn into
small pieces 2 teaspoons of prepared yellow mustard
1 tablespoon Splenda pourable or Sugar Twin
1 teaspoon dried parsley flakes
1 cup (an 8-ounce can) Hunt's Tomato Sauce

Spray a slow cooker container with a butter-flavoured cooking spray. In a large bowl, combine meat, onion, bread pieces, mustard and a second cup of tomato sauce. Mix well to combine. Form it in a large ball. Place in a prepared slow cooker container. Stir the Splenda flakes and parsley into the remaining tomato sauce and the spoon mixture evenly over the meatloaf. Cover and cook on LOW for 6 to 8 hours. Divide into 8 servings. When ready to serve, spoon evenly of sauce on top.

Serves 8,167 cal, 7 fat gm, 17 gm pro, 9 gm carbohydrates, , 340 mg turf, 18 mg calcium, 1 gm fiber

Chicken Paprika slow Cooker in wine
Makes 4 servings

1/2 cup dry white wine 2
tsp olive oil
1 lb boneless, skinless chicken breast, cut into fat and cut into 4 p.m. 1 tsp cumin
seeds
1 tsp mustard seeds
4 garlic cloves, finely chopped
1 tbsp. Paprika
1 large onion, thinly sliced
4 oz mushrooms, sliced parsley
sprigs to garnish
Rings of sweet red pepper, to garnish

Pour the wine into the pot. Heat 1 tbsp of oil in a frying pan, and brown chicken on both sides over low heat, 3-5 min. Transfer chicken to pot, and sprinkle over cumin, mustard, garlic and paprika. Add the remaining oil to the same skillet and fry the onions and mushrooms until lightly browned, 2-3 min. Pour over chicken. Cover and cook on LOW until chicken is tender, 7 to 9 hours. Garnish with parsley and peppers.

Per serving: 268 cal, 7g fat, 1.5g sat fat, 96 mg   chol, 89 mg turf, 1.3g fib

Slow-cook pierogies **with Pepper-Shallot sauce**
Hommes 6 portions Grand Pot de crockery

1 can (28 oz) crushed tomatoes
1 shallot, thinly sliced
1 cup sweet green peppers, chopped 1/2
teaspoon olive oil
1/2 tbsp red wine vinegar
1/2 tsp Italian herb seasoning 1/2
teaspoon black pepper
1 lb deterre pierogies filled withde potatoes, fresh or frozen (thawed)

Mix the first 7 ingredients in the pot. Cover and cook on LOW for 5-9 hours. or on HIGH for 3 1/2 to 5 hours. Add the pierogies. Cover and cook for 1 hour. Per serving: 179 cal,, 2.1 g fat, 0.7 g sat fat, 10 mg   chol,, 522 mg turf, 4.2 g fib

Slow cooker pork roast with creamy mustard sauce
Makes 8 servings

2 boneless boneless boneless boneless pork sirloin roast 2 1/2-3 lbs
1 tbsp vegetable oil 3/4
cup dry white wine 2 tbsp
all-purpose flour 1 tsp.
Salt
1/2 teaspoon pepper
Two med. carrots, finely chopped or grated
1 m. onion, finely chopped (1/2 cup)
1 small shallot, finely chopped
(2tbsp)1/4cup half and a half
2 to 3 tbsp Dijon mustard in the countryside

Cut off excess pork fat. Heat oil in 10-inch skillet over low heat. Cook the pork in oil for about 10 min., turning occasionally, until brown on all sides. Place pork in 3 1/2-6 qt. slow cooker. Mix remaining ingredients except for half and mustard; pour over the pork. Cover and cook on LOW 7-9 hours. or until the pork is tender. Remove pork from stove; cover and keep warm. Cut the fat from pork juice in the stove, if desired. Stir half and half and mustard in juices. Cover and cook on HIGH for about 15 min. or until slightly thickened. Serve the sauce with pork.

Per serving: cal 175, fat 9g, fat sat 3g, chol 55mg, turf 390mg, carbohydrates 5g, fib 1g, prot 20g

Slow cookery salmon patties
Makes 4 servings (1 patty each)

2 large eggs, fork beaten
2.75 oz salmon, drained, round skin and bones removed 1/2 cup
water
1 cup soda cracker crumbs 1/2
teaspoon celery salt
1/2 teaspoon onion
powder 1/4 teaspoon
salt
1/4 tsp diced dill
1/16 teaspoon.
1/2 cup corn flake breadcrumbs

Mix the first 9 ingredients in a bowl. Shape into 8 patties. Coat with cornflake breadcrumbs. Place 4 patties on the bottom of a slow 3 1/2 or 5 qt stove. Place the remaining patties on top. Cover. **Cook at low** hours for 4-5 hours or on HIGH for **2 to 2 -1/2 hours.**

Per serving: 171cal, 7.7 g fat, 578 mg turf, 11 g prot,13 g carbohydrates

Slow Cooker Salsa Swiss Steak

Makes 5 servings

2 tsp oil
1 1/2 lbs boneless round beef steak, cut into fat, cut into 5 pc. 1/2 teaspoon salt
1/4 teaspoon pepper
1 onion i0dic, halved lengthwise, sliced
1/2 med. green pepper, cut into bite strips
1 (10 3/4 oz) can condensed cream of mushroom soup 3/4
cup thick and stocky salsa

Heat oil in a large skillet over hot heat until hot. Sprinkle steak with salt and pepper. Put the steak in the pan, cook for 4-6 min. or until golden brown, turning once. Transfer steak to a slow cooker for 4 to 6 qt. Garnish with onion and pepper. In the same skillet, combine soup and salsa; mix well. Pour over vegetables and steak. Cover; cook on LOW for 8-10 hours.

Remove steak pieces from slow cooker; place on the serving tray. Mix the sauce well and serve with the steak. Per serving: cal 260, fat 11g, fat sat 3g, chol 70mg, carbohydrates 10g, fib 1g, prot 30g

Dinner slow cooker-sausage and sauerkraut

Makes 4 servings (2 cups)

6 small red potatoes, unpeeled, in quarters
8 fresh carrots, cut into 1/4-inch slices
1 med. onion, cut into thin wedges
1 tbsp brown sugar
1 tbsp spicy brown mustard
1 tsp caraway seeds
1 (15 oz) can sauerkraut
1 lb fully cooked turkey kielbasa, cut into 1-inch slices

In 3 1/2-4 qt. mixpotatoes, carrots and onion. In the med bowl. , combine brown sugar, mustard and caraway seeds; mix well. Stir in sauerkraut and kielbasa. Pour the sauerkraut mixture over the vegetables in a cookery. Cover; cook on LOW for at least 8 hours. or until the vegetables are tender.

Per serving: cal 360, fat 7g, fat sat 1g, chol 70mg, turf 2040mg, carbohydrates 51g, fib 7g, sug 8g, prot 13g

Slow Cooker scalloped potatoes

6 m2 potatoes (2 lbs), cut into 1/8-inch slices
1 can (10 3/4oz) condensed onion soup cream 1 can (5
oz) evaporated milk (2/3 cup)
1 jar (2 oz) diced pimientos, not dedraded
1/2teaspoons. Salt
1/4 teaspoon pepper

Spray inside 3 1/2-6 qt. slow cooker with a cooking spray. Mix all ingredients; ingrédients; pour into the stove. Cover and cook on LOW 10-12 hours. or until the potatoes are tender. Makes 8 servings

Par portion: cal 155 , gras 3 g , sat gras 1 g , cho 10 mg , sod 460 mg , carb 30 g , fib 2 g , prot 4 g

Potatoes and ham scallops simmered

6 cups frozen grated potatoes (Ore Ida Hash Browns (Southern Style) Fat Free - 32 oz bag). 1 cup peas, frozen
1 1/2 cups Ham, extra lean - diced
1 1/2 cups cheddar cheese, Kraft Reduced Fat - grated
1 can of mushroom soup cream, condensed, healthy demand 2/3 cup
non-greasy dry milk powder
1 cup water
1/4 cup onion - diced 1
tsp dried parsley

In a slow cooker, combine potatoes, peas, ham and cheddar cheese. In a medium bowl, combine mushroom soup, dry milk powder, water, onion and parsley flakes. Add soup mixture to potato mixture. Mix well to combine. Cover and cook over low heat for 6 to 8 hours.

264 Calories; 8 gm Fat; 19 gm Pr;29 gm Ca;732 mg So; 320 mg Cl;3 gm Fi. (Serve 1 cup)

Scalloped potatoes and slow cooker turkey
Makes 6 servings (1 1/4 cups)

1 lb ground turkey breast 1/2
teaspoon ground thyme
1/8 tsp pepper 1 (7.8 oz) Hungry Jack Cheesy Scalloped potatoes 2 tbsp
margarine or butter
2 1/2 cups boiling water
1 1/2 cups skimmed milk
1 med. red pepper, seeded, chopped
1 med. onion,thinly sliced

Spray a large frying pan with a non-stick spray. Heat over low heat until hot. Add ground turkey, cook until golden and no longer pink. Stir in thyme and pepper. In a large bowl, combine sauce from pkg., potato slices and margarine. Add boiling water; stir until margarine melts. Add milk; mix well. Stir in browned turkey, pepper and onion.

Pour the mixture into a slow 3 1/2 or 4 qt stove. With the back of the spoon, squeeze the potatoes to cover with sauce. Cover; cook on LOW for at least 7 hours. or until the potatoes are tender.

Per serving: cal 290, fat 7g, fat sat 2g, chol 45mg, turf 780mg, carbohydrates 34g, fib 2g, prot 27g

Slow Cooker Sloppy Joes
Makes 24 sandwiches

3 lbs ground beef
1 large onion, coarsely chopped 3/4
cup chopped celery
1 cup barbecue sauce
1 can (26 1/2 oz) sloppy joe sauce
24 hamburger buns

Bake beef and onion in Oven in The Oven, stirring occasionally, until beef is brown; Aspire. Mix the beef mixture and the rest of the ingredients, except the buns in a slow 3 1/2 to 6 qt cookery.
Cover and cook low for 7-9 hours. (orou HIGH 3 to 4 hours.) or until the vegetables are tender. Uncover and cook on HIGH until desired consistency. Stir well before serving. Fill buns with beef mixture.

Per sandwich; cal cal 155, fat 9g, fat sat 3g, chol 30mg, turf 270mg, carb 8g, fib 1g, prot 11g

Slow Cooker Steak Burritos
Makes 10 servings

2 flank steaks (about 1 lb each)
2 taco seasoning envelopes with reduced sodium content
1 med. onion,chopped
1 can (4 oz) chopped green peppers
1 tbsp vinegar
10 fat-free flour tortillas (7inches)1 1/2 cups (6 oz(grated Montery Jack cheese reduced in fat 1
1/2 cup chopped plum tomatoes
3/4 cup non-greasy sour cream

Cut steaks in half; rub with taco seasoning. Place in a slow cooker coated with non-stick spray. Garnish with onion, chillies and vinegar. Cover and cook on LOW for 8 to 9 hours. or until the meat is tender. Remove steaks and allow to cool slightly; shred the meat with 2 forks. Return to slow cooker; heat through. Pour about 1/2 cup of meat mixture into the centre of each tortilla. Garnish with cheese, tomato and sour cream. Fold the ends and sides over the filling.

Per serving: 339 cal, 580mg turf, 57mg chol,31g carbohydrates, 28g prot,10g fat, 2g fibre

Slow cooker stew

16 ounces lean beef stew, cubed into one
and two cups chopped onion
2 cups chopped carrots
1 1/2 cups chopped celery
4 cups diced raw potatoes
1 3/4 cup (a 15-ounce can) Swanson Beef Broth 1
tablespoon parsley flakes
1/2 teaspoon Italian seasoning 1/8
teaspoon black pepper
2 tablespoons Quick Cooking Minute
Tapioca

In a large frying pan sprayed with butter-flavoured cooking spray, brown the meat with stew. Spray a slow cooker container with cooking spray. Place the browned meat in a prepared container. Add onion, carrots, celery and potatoes. Mix well to combine. In a small bowl, combine beef broth, parsley flakes, Italian seasoning, black pepper and uncooked tapioca. Pour the mixture over the vegetables. Cover and coon on LOW for 8 hours. Mix well before serving. Serves 6 (1 1/2 cups)

Sweet and sour slow cooker pork

Service size 4

1 1/2 pounds pork loins, lean, boneless - cubed
8 ounces canned pineapple pieces in juice -- un bronchial (unsweetened juice) 1
medium red pepper -- cut into squares or green pepper bronzés
3 tablespoons brown sugar w/Brown Sugar Twin or Splenda, CarolTM 1/2 teaspoon
ginger
1/4 cup vinegar
3 tablespoons soy sauce
3 tablespoons water
2 tablespoons cornstarch
2 cups cooked rice

In a slow cooker of 3-1/2 to 4 liters, combine pork, pineapple, pepper, brown sugar, ginger, vinegar and soy sauce. Mix well. Cover; cook on the LOW setting for 6 to 8 hours. About 5 minutes before serving, in a small bowl, mix 3 tablespoons of water and cornstarch; maïs; mix well. Stir pork mixture into a slow cooker. Cover; cook over high heat for an additional 5 minutes or until thickened. Serve pork mixture over rice. Prepare the rice 25 minutes before serving.

Per serving (excluding unknown items): 410 calories; 8g fat (17.4% calories from fat); 34g protein; 49g carbohydrates; 2g dietary fibre; 77mg Cholesterol; 841mg sodium.
Rice is counted on the total.

Tasty slow cooker mex casserole

Makes 10 servings (1 cup)

1 1/2 lbs lean ground beef
3 tbsp white vinegar
1 tbsp chili powder
1 tsp dried whole oregano 1/4
teaspoon garlic powder
1 1/2 teaspoons
salt 1/4 teaspoon
pepper
1 1/4 cups chopped onion
1 med. green pepper, chopped
4 oz canned chopped green peppers, drained (optional)
12 oz canned whole corn, drained
1 cup macaroni at the elbow, partially cooked, drained and rinsed
2 (14 oz) cans of tomatoes with juice, broken
2 tsp chili powder
1 tsp parsley flakes
1/2 tsp dried whole oregano 2 tsp
granulated sugar
1/2 teaspoon salt
1/4 teaspoon
pepper

Mix the first 7 ingredients in a bowl. Fry in a non-stick frying pan until golden. Aspire. Put the onion in 3 1/2 or 5 qt. slow cooker. Add green pepper, green peppers, corn and partially cooked macaroni. Add beef mixture. Stir. Mix the remaining 7 ingredients in a bowl. Stir well. Pour over top. Stir. Cover. Cook on LOW for 8 hours. or on HIGH for 4 hours.

Per serving: 206cal, 6.5 g fat, 874 mg turf, 16 g prot,23 g carbohydrates

Minestrone of slow cooker vegetables

4 cups vegetable or chicken broth

4 cups tomato juice
1 tablespoon dried basil leaves
1 teaspoon salt
1/2 teaspoon dried oregano leaves 1/4
teaspoon pepper
2 medium carrots - sliced (1 cup)
2 medium celery stalks, chopped (1 cup)
1 medium onion, chopped (1/2 cup)
1 cup sliced fresh mushrooms (3 ounces)
2 garlic cloves - finely chopped
1 can diced tomatoes (28 ounces) unsplupped - 1 1/2
cups raw rotini pasta - 4 1/2 ounces grated Parmesan
cheese if desired

Mix all ingredients in a 4 to 5 litre slow cooker, except pasta and cheese. Cover and cook over low heat for 7 to 8 hours or until vegetables are tender. Stir in pasta, cover and cook over high heat for 15 to 20 minutes or until pasta is tender. Sprinkle each serving with cheese.

Slow Cooker Wild Rice Soup

1/2 cup wild rice - 1/2 cup
grated carrot
3 cans fat-free chicken broth
1 Boneless skinless chicken breast tote -- cut into 1 1/2-inch pieces of chopped
celery -- about 1 stalk
1/2 cup chopped onion -- about 1 medium onion 8 ounces
spinach leaves, whole
1 cup fat-free sour cream 1/2
cup flour

Combine all ingredients except spinach, sour cream and flour in a slow cooker. Cover; cook on LOW for 10-12 hours. or until the chicken and rice are tender. Just before serving, mix sour cream and flour in a small bowl until smooth. Increase heat to HIGH. Add spinach and slowly mix sour cream mixture into hot soup mixture, stirring constantly. Cook, stirring occasionally, until soup is thickened and creamy (6 to 10 min.).

Yield:"8 Cups" per serving: 165 Calories (kcal); 1 g total fat; 22g protein; 20g carbohydrates; 36mg Cholesterol; 272mg sodium

Slow Cooker Spicy Black-Eyed Peas

Makes 8 servings

1 lb black-eyed dried peas (2 cups),
sorted and rinsed
1 med. onion,chopped (1/2 cup)
6 cups water
1 tsp salt
1/2 teaspoon pepper
3/4 cup med. or hot salsa

Mix all ingredients except salsa in 3 1/2 qt. à 6 qt. slow cooker. Cover and cook over high heat for 3 to 4 hours. or until the peas are tender. Stir in salsa. Cover and cook on HIGH for about 10 min or until hot.

Per serving: cal 145,fat 1g, sitting fat 0g, chol 0mg, turf 360mg, carb 35g, fibre 11g, prot 13g

Smoky Ham et Navy Bean Stew

1 pound extra lean ham -- cut into 1/2-inch (3 cup) cubes -see note 2
cups water
1 cup dried sea beans
1 cup sliced celery

2 medium carrots -- sliced
1/4 teaspoon dried thyme leaves

1/4 teaspoon salting liquid smoke 1/4 cup
chopped fresh parsley

Note: I used extra lean ham he called for cooked ham. I believe they used extra lean cooked ham according to nutritional values.

In 3-1/2 to 4 quarters of slow cooker, combine all ingredients except parsley; mix well. Cover and cook at low setting for 10 to 12 hours. Just before serving, stir in parsley.

4 servings (1-1/4 cups). Yield: "5 cups"

Per serving: 345 calories; 6g fat; 34g protein; 38g carbohydrates; 14g dietary fibre; 53mg cholesterol; 1675mg sodium.

Service suggestion: Crispy French rolls and butter with a glass of wine, as well as a fruit crisp topped with whipped cream.

NOTES: Please note the dry beans, I covered with water brought to a boil and boiled for 5 minutes. He removed the fire and let it soak all night.

Smoky Joe Slow-Cooker Beef Stew

1 pound well-stocked beef cubes
3/4 cup drained salsa and barbecue sauce
1 packet (1.25 ounces) reduced to sodium taco seasoning mixture
2 cups frozen corn
2 cans (15 ounces) rinsed and drained of black beans
1 (19 ounces) can rinse and drain chickpeas or garbanzo beans 1/2 cup
fresh coriander

In a 3-quarter or 4-quarter slow cooker, combine beef, salsa, barbecue sauce, taco mixture and corn; mix well. Cover and cook for 3 to 4 hours or 6 to 8 hours, or until meat is tender. Add beans and coriander; mix well. Cover and let stand for 5 minutes so that the beans heat up.

Provides 8 nutritional information per serving: 301 calories; 23g protein; 5g fat; 40g carbohydrates; 35mg cholesterol; 1,002 mg sodium; 11g fibre.

Smothered chicken

4 skinless whole skinless chicken breasts without skin
12 ounces mushrooms -- fresh
1 can 98% fat-free Mushroom Soup Cream 1 can 98% fat-free Chicken soup cream
1 can French celery onion
soup -- chopped or baby
corn -- etc.

Cut chicken breasts into stew-sized pieces and sauté while washing and cutting mushrooms in half. Then just add all the ingredients to the chicken and simmer for about 1 hour. You can also do this in a simmering pot all day until dinner. Serve over rice, noodles or potatoes.

Per serving: 280 calories; 3g fat; 56g protein; 4g carbohydrates; 1g dietary fibre; 137mg Cholesterol; 161mg sodium.

Smothered chicken with pierogies
Serves 4

1 dozen frozen potatoes and Pierogies Cheddar Cheese 1 can (10 3/4 oz)low-fat cream of chicken soup
1 can (4oz) sliced mushrooms, drained
1 cup frozen peas
2 cups cubed or grated chicken

Preheat the oven to 350 years and older. Spray a 2-quarter saucepan with non-stick coating. Thaw the Pierogies in boiling water for 5 minutes, drain and place in the pan. In a large saucepan, combine soup, mushrooms, peas and chicken. Cook, stirring, for about 5 minutes or until hot. Pour over Pierogies. Bake for 15 minutes.

Smothered steak
Makes 6 servings

1 (1 1/2 lbs) lean boneless round steak
3 tbsp all-purpose flour
1/4 teaspoon.
1 (14 1/2 oz) pkg. frozen chopped onion, celery and pepper mixture, thawed
2 tbs. Worcestershire low-sodium sauce
1 tbs. red wine vinegar
1/4 tsp salt
3 cooked cups long grain rice (cooked without salt or fat)

Cut steak fat; Cut steak into 1 1/2-inch pcs. Place steak in 4 tt electric slow cooker. Add flour and pepper; poivre; Throw. Add tomato and the following 4 ingredients and mix well. Cover and cook on HIGH 1hour.;

reduce heat to LOW and cook for 7 hours. or until steak is tender, stirring once.

To serve, pour evenly more than one/2 cup of rice.
Per serving: cal 312, fat 5.1g, fat sat 1.8g, prot 27.9g, carbohydrates 36.5g, fibre 0.6g, chol 68mg, turf 225mg

Lasagna south of the border
Makes 7-8 servings

3/4 lb turkey sausage
2 tomatoes, seeded and chopped
3 fresh tomatillos, inked and chopped
1 (19 oz) peut sauce enchilada verte
1 clove garlic, crushed
1/4 teaspoon salt
1/8 tsp ground black pepper 8 oz
lasagna noodles
1 cup low-fat or fat-free ricotta cheese
1 cup freshly grated chopped chopped coriander cheese

Crumble the sausage in a slow cooker. Stir in tomatoes, tomatillos, enchilada sauce, garlic, salt and pepper. Cover and cook at low 5 1/2 to 6 hours.

Preheat the oven to 350 euros Grease a 13x9 baking dish. Cook the lasagna noodles according to the pkg directions. and drain. Spread about 1/2 cup of turkey mixture in the bottom of the prepared pan; have extra layers of noodles, ricotta cheese and hot turkey mixture. Garnish with Jack cheese. Bake for 25 to 30 minutes or until boiling around the edges. Sprinkle with coriander.

Per serving: Cal 340 - Carb 36 g - Prot 21 g - Total fat 13 g - Sat fat 3 g - Cal fat 117 - Chol 56 mg - Sodium 817 mg

Southwest bean stew with cornmeal dumplings
Makes 4 servings

1 15 oz can red beans, rinsed and drained
1 15 oz can black beans, pinto beans, or large northern beans, rinsed and drained 3 cups water
1 14-1/2 oz Mexican-style simmered tomatoes
1 10 oz package frozen whole corn, thawed 2 medium
carrots, sliced (1 cup)
1 large onion, chopped (1 cup)
1 4 oz chopped green peppers
2 tsp instant beef or chicken broth granules or 2 cubes of vegetable stock 1 to 2 tsp chili powder
2 garlic cloves, chopped 1/3
cup all-purpose flour 1/4
cup yellow cornmeal 1 tsp
Salt dash baking powder
Dash pepper
1 egg white, beaten
2 Tbs. Lait
1 Tbs. cooking oil

In 3-1/1/2 or 4-quarter electric dishes, combine canned beans, water, tomatoes, corn, carrots, onion, non-soft peppers,, broth granules or cubes, chili powder and garlic. Cover and cook over low heat for 10 to 12 hours or set at high temperature for 4 to 5 hours.

For the meatballs, in a small mixing bowl, combine flour, cornmeal, baking powder, salt and pepper. In another small mixing bowl, combine egg white, milk and cooking oil. Add the white egg mixture to the flour mixture; stir with a fork until smooth. If the stew is cooked over low heat, turn the dishtop in a high heat setting. Place the meatball mixture in 8 teaspoons rounded at the top of the stew. Cover; cook for another 30 minutes (do not lift the lid).

Per serving: 391 cal., 6 g fat (1 g fat), 1 mg chol., 1,471 mg sodium, 77 g carbo.,12 g fiber, 22 g pro.

Southwest Chicken Chili

1 medium green pepper, chopped
1 cup chopped onions
3 garlic cloves, chopped
3 tablespoons cornmeal
2 tablespoons chili powder
3 teaspoons dried oregano leaves
1 teaspoon cumin
1 teaspoon salt
1 1/4 Pounds boneless skinless chicken thighs - cut into 1" pieces 1 Jar 16
Oz. sauce medium picting sauce
1 15 Oz Can pinto haricots - non-dédracés
1 14,5 Oz Can Diced Tomatoes - nondrained

In a slow 3 1/2 to 4 litre cooker, combine pepper, onion and garlic. In a medium bowl, combine corn flour, chili powder, oregano, cumin and salt; mix well. Add chicken; toss to coat. Add chicken and remaining vegetable seasoning mixture to slow cooker. Add the pickening sauce, beans and tomatoes; stir gently to mix. Cook at low setting for 6-8 hours.

For a more spicy chilli, use 3 tablespoons of chili powder. For a less spicy recipe, use sweet pickening sauce or salsa.

Yield: "1 1/3 Cups" Per serving (NOTES: 280 cal., 8 g. fat, 60 mg chol., 1330 mg. turf., 29 g. carbohydrates, 7 g.fiber,5 g. sugars 1 1/2 starch, 1 veg., 2 lean meat, 1/2 fat

Southwest Meatloaf

Vegetable cooking spray
2 lb brown ground (I used 93% lean ground beef) 3 slices
light bread, crumbled (1 cup)
1 cup chopped onion (about 1 medium) 1/2
cup fat-free egg substitute
1/4 teaspoon salt
1/4 teaspoon ground pepper
1/2 cup ketchup
1/2 cup thick, chunky salsa (I used chili sauce)

Coat 3 slow cookers with a quarter and a quarter of a spray. Wrap two lengths of aluminum foil long enough to fit in the bottom of the stove and extend 3 inches on each side of the stove. Fold each strip of aluminum foil lengthwise to form 2-inch-wide strips. Arrange the foil strips in a cross-framed manner in the stove, pressing the strip in the bottom of the stove and extending the ends to the sides of the stove. Mix beef and the following 5 ingredients; shape the mixture into bread in the shape of the slow cooker container. Place the bread in the slow cooker over the foil strips. (The aluminum foil strips become "handles" to remove the meatloaf from the slow cooker.) Make a shallow indention on top of the meatloaf. Mix ketchup and salsa (chili sauce);); pour over the meatloaf. Cover and cook over low heat for 8 hours or over high heat for 3 1/2 to 4 hours. Use strips of aluminum foil to lift the meatloaf from the stove. Let the meatloaf rest for 10 minutes before serving.

Yield: 8 servings. 209 calories;9.8g carbohydrate;6.0g fat;1.1g fiber;27.9g protein; 66mg cholesterol; 415 mg sodium; 31mg calcium;3.1mg iron.

Southwest Slow cooker slow cooker soup

3/4 LB(s) boneless, skinless chicken breast, cut into 1-inch cubes 3 small sweet
potatoes, or 2 medium, peeled and cut into 1-inch cubes 1 large onions,
chopped
29 oz   canned diced tomatoes, salsa-style with   chillies, nondrained 14
1/2 oz fat-free chicken broth
1 tsp dried oregano 1/2
tsp ground cumin
1 1/2 cups (s) frozen corn kernels, not thawed

Combine chicken, potatoes, onion, tomatoes, broth, oregano and cumin in a slow cooker of 4-quarters or more (crockpot);); cover and cook over low heat for at least 6 hours. Stir in corn; cover and cook over high heat until chicken is no longer pink in centre and vegetables are tender, about 30 minutes. Makes about 1 1/4 cups per serving. For Lesservant 4

Hunter de poulet spécial

1 cup (an 8-ounce can) tomatoes, finely chopped andundinged 1 (10 3/4
ounces) can Healthy Demand Tomato Soup
1 1/2 teaspoon Italian seasonings 1/2
teaspoon dried chopped garlic
1/2 cup (one 2.5 ounce jar) sliced mushrooms, drained 1/2
cup chopped green pepper
1/2 cup chopped onion
16 ounces peeled and boneless chicken breast, cut into 4 pieces

In a slow cooker container sprayed with olive oil flavoured cooking spray, combine unredging,   tomatoes, tomato soup, Italian seasoning and garlic. Stir in mushrooms, green pepper and onion. Add chicken pieces. Mix well to combine. Cover and cook on LOW for 6 to 8 hours. When ready to serve, spoon evenly of sauce over the chicken.

Yields 4 equal portions: 204 Calories - 4 fat gm - 25 proteins gm   -   17 gm Carbohydrates - 531 mg sodium - 29 mg calcium - 2 gm Fiber

Spicy wine pot roast
3-pound beef pot roast
1 small onion, chopped
1 mixture of brown sauce with packaging
1 cup water
1/4 cup ketchup
1/4 cup dry red wine
2 teaspoons Dijon-style mustard
1 teaspoon Worcestershire sauce 1/8
teaspoon garlic powder
1/2 teaspoon Italian seasoning dried Salt
Freshly ground black pepper
Fresh parsley - to garnish, - chopped

Sprinkle the meat with salt and pepper. Place in slow cooker. Mix the rest of the ingredients, except the parsley, and pour over the meat. Cover and cook low for 10 hours. Remove meat and slice. Thicken the sauce with flour mixed in a small amount of water and serve on the meat sprinkled with chopped parsley.

Serving size (1/12 recipe) Per serving: 252.6 calories, 17.8 g fat, 0.3 g fibre

Stir-Fry Lo Mein
Makes 6 servings

2 tbsp butter
1 (20 oz pkg) boneless skinless chicken thighs, cut into bite-sized pcs. 1 cup sautéed seasoned sauce)cuisses
1 (5 oz) can water chestnuts, drained
1 med. (1/2 cup) onion, sliced
1 (16 oz) pkg fresh sautéed vegetables (celery, carrots, broccoli and pea pods) 1/2 cup whole cashew nuts (optional)
1 (8 oz) pkg. lo mine noodles

Melt the butter in a 10-inch skillet until sizzling; add chicken pcs. Cook over low-cold heat, turning occasionally, until chicken is golden brown (5 to 7 min.) Place in slow cooker. Add sautéed seasoning sauce, water chestnuts and onion. Cover; cook on setting on low heat for 4-6 hours. Increase heat setting to HIGH 30 minutes before serving. Add sautéed vegetables; Stir. Cover; cook for 30 minutes, stirring once, until vegetables are tenderly crisp. Stir in cashew nuts just before serving, if desired. Meanwhile, cook the noodles lo mine according to the pkg directions. To serve, pour chicken and sautéed vegetables mixture over noodles.

Per serving: cal 430, pro 28g, carb 52g, 5g fibre, 13g fat, 90mg chol, turf 1790mg
This can be done with frozen sautéed vegetables. Increase the heat setting to HIGH and cook for 45 minutes to 1 hour until the vegetables are tender.

Stuffed beef rolls

1 1/2 lb Top Round Steak -- 1/2 inch thick. 4 slices of bacon reduced in fat
3/4 cup celery -- diced
3/4 cup onion -- diced
1/2 cup green pepper -- diced 10 ounces beef sauce
Garlic powder to taste - if desired.

Cut steak into four equal-sized pieces. Sprinkle lightly with garlic powder. Place a slice of bacon on each piece of meat. Combine celery, onion and green pepper in medium bowl; place about 1/2 cup of mixture on each piece of meat. Roll the meat; secured ends with wooden toothpicks. Place on a paper towel to absorb any extra meat juices. Place steak buns in a simmering jar. Pour sauce evenly over steak rolls to moisten. Cover the crock-pot and cook over low heat for 8 to 10 hours or high for 4 to 5 hours. Cut off any grease before serving.

Per serving: 254 calories; 13g fat; 28g protein; 5g carbohydrates; 1g dietary fibre; 58mg cholesterol; 501mg sodium.

Pasta shells stuffed with mushroom sauce

Donne 6 portions Grand Crockery Pot

8 oz mushrooms, sliced
2 tsp olive oil
2 soy-sausage patties (or regular sausages for breakfast)
1 can (28 oz) plum tomatoes, cut
1 can (6 oz) low-sodium tomato paste 1/2
teaspoon dried oregano
1/2 teaspoon garlic
powder 1/2 cup dry white
wine
1 pkg. (20 oz) low-fat cheese stuffed pasta shells
Snipped fresh Italian parsley, to garnish

Sauté mushrooms in oil in a non-stick skillet, until golden, about 5 min. Transfer to pot. In the same skillet, cook sausage patties for 6 minutes. Remove them from the pan and cut into a quarter-inch cubes. Place the pcs. in the dishwashing jar. Stir in tomatoes, tomato paste, oregano, garlic and wine. Cover and cook over high heat for 3 and a half hours. Add the shells to the sauce, making sure to cover with sauce. Cover and cook until shells are hot, about 1 hour. Garnish with parsley.

Per serving: 212 cal, 6.9g fat, 1.9g sat fat, 8.3 mg chol, 584 mg turf, 3.4g fib

Sunday Italian Vegetable Soup

1/2 cup dry beans of sea
water
4 cups chicken broth
3/4 cup carrot -- sliced, peeled 1/2
cup potato -- sliced with zest 1
tablespoon corn oil
1/2 cup onion -- sliced
2 cups canned Italian tomatoes -non-deed
2 cups cabbage - thinly sliced
1 cup zucchini -- sliced 1/2
cup celery -- sliced
1/2 cup canned chickpeas -- (garbanzo beans)- drained in can 1/2 cup
Rotini or other pasta -- uncooked
1 tablespoon fresh parsley - finely chopped fresh
2 teaspoons dried basil - crumbled 1/4
teaspoon salt
1/4 teaspoon ground pepper - fresh

Cover the sea beans with water in a large saucepan. Over medium heat, bring just to a boiling point. Remove the pan from the heat, cover and let stand for 1 hour. Aspire. Add chicken broth, carrot and potato. Cover and cook over medium heat until vegetables are almost tender, about 35 minutes. Heat the oil in a small frying pan and fry the onion until tender. Add the onion and all the remaining ingredients to the soup. Bake for 15 minutes or until pasta is cooked. Serve hot.

Per serving: 212 calories; 4g fat; 11g protein; 34g carbohydrates; 9g dietary fibre; 0mg Cholesterol; 862mg sodium.

Souper Potluck Potluck

16 ounces ground 90% lean turkey or beef
3 cups (15 ounces) sliced raw potatoes
1-1/2 cups chopped celery
2 cups sliced carrots
1 cup chopped onion
1-1/2 cups frozen peas
2 teaspoons Italian seasoning
1-3/4 cups (a 15-ounce can) Chunky Hunt's Tomato Sauce

In a large frying pan sprayed with a butter-flavoured cooking spray, brown meat. Meanwhile, place potatoes, celery, carrots and onion in Crock-Pot container. Sprinkle the peas on top. Pour the browned meat over the vegetables. Stir in Italian seasoning with tomato sauce. Pour the sauce evenly over the meat. Cover. Cook on LOW 6 to 8 hours. Stir well just before serving.

258 Calories; 8 fats; 18 gm proteins; ; 29 gm carbohydrates; ; 559 mg sodium; 4 gm 6 fibers (1-1/4 cups)

Soft and sour wings

3 pounds of chicken wings -- (about 28 pieces of wings) or 18 drumettes 1
cup packaged brown sugar
1/4 cup all-purpose flour
1/2 cup water
1/4 cup white vinegar
1 1/2 tablespoons ketchup 1/4
cup soy sauce
1/4 teaspoon garlic powder 1
tablespoon onion flakes 1/2
teaspoon salt
1/2 teaspoon prepared mustard

Discard the tip and cut the wings at the joint. Place chicken pieces in a 5-litre slow cooker. Mix brown sugar and flour well in a saucepan. Add water, vinegar and ketchup. Stir. Add the remaining 5 ingredients. Heat and stir until boiling and thickened. Pour over the wings. Cover. Cook on LOW for 8 or 9 hours or on HIGH for 4 to 4 and a half hours until tender. Serve from a slow cooker or solvent on a tray. Makes 28 wing pieces or about 18 drumettes....

Per serving (excluding unknown items): 95 calories; 4g fat; 5g protein; 9g carbohydrates; dietary fibre trace; 20mg cholesterol; 218mg sodium.
I usually buy wings that are already separated and bits removed.

Sweet and sour meat and rice

16 oz   extra lean ground turkey or beef
1 cup crushed pineapple, wrapped in fruit juice, not flaked
1 3/4 cups tomato sauce
2 C. Brown sugar soup
1 tbsp reduced sodium soy sauce
1 1/2 cups chopped green pepper
1 cup chopped onion
2 tsp dried parsley flakes
1 1/3 cups uncooked instant rice

In a large frying pan sprayed with a butter-flavoured cooking spray, brown meat. Spray a slow cooker container with butter-flavoured spray. In a prepared undrained container, combine undracerated pineapple, tomatosauce, brown sugar and soy sauce. Stir in green pepper, onion and parsley flakes. Add browned meat and raw rice. Mix well to combine. Cover and cook over low heat for 6 hours. Mix well before serving.

Serves 6 (1 cup)
239 Calories, 7 grmfats, 16 gm proteins, , 28 gmcarbohydrates, 587 mg sodium, 31 mg calcium, 3 gm fibers. .

Sweet and spicy chicken "DUMP"

1 Package Taco Seasoning Mix
8 oz   apricot jam
12 oz Salsa
1 1/2 pounds of chicken pieces

For immediate cooking: Preheat the oven to 350 F. Place all the ingredients in a large ovenproof dish, process the coated chicken. Bake until chicken juice is clear (45-60 minutes for chicken pieces, or 20-30 minutes for chicken breasts).

For freezing: Place all ingredients in a 1-gallon freezer bag. Place flat in the freezer.
To thaw and cook: Remove the bag from the freezer the day before, make sure the bag is completely closed. Place the bag on a shelf furthest from the freezer (it's best if the bag is laid   flat, although it may not be the best option with a refrigerator/freezer side by side). Preheat the oven to 350 F. Empty the contents of the bag into a large ovenproof dish and bake until the juice is clear (45-60 minutes for the chicken pieces, or 20-30 minutes for the chicken breasts). For the slow cooker: Put the chicken in the bottom of the pan, pour over the remaining ingredients (mixed) and cook until the chicken is cooked! IT'S SIMPLE!

Swiss chicken casserole
1 portion

1 packet of pan top stuffing mixture
4-6 boneless/skinless chicken breasts
4 slices Swiss cheese
1 can of low-fat cream of mushroom soup

Take 1 packet of pan top stuffing mixture and mix the two dry packages together. Don't add any water yet. Place in a spray slow cooker (with Pam). Place boneless, skinless chicken breasts 4-6 on top of stuffing. Place the Swiss cheese on top of the chicken, then spread the reduced cream of mushroom soup over the chicken and cheese. Spread evenly. Water 1/4 - 1/2 cup of hot water at the edges. Cook over low heat in a slow cooker all day. If you don't use or have a slow cooker, you can bake it in the oven at 350 degrees for an hour.

Swiss steak #2

1 1/2 lbs round beef steak (1/2 inch thick), cut into portion-sized pcs. 2 cups sliced onions
1 (4.5 oz) whole pot mushrooms, drained
1 (10 3/4 oz) can condensed beef broth 1/4 teaspoon salt
1/4 teaspoon pepper 1/4 cup water
2 tbsp cornstarch

Heat the oven to 325 euros. In a large ovenproof skillet, a Dutch oven or an ovenproof dish, combine all ingredients except water and cornstarch; mix well. Cover. Bake at 325 and a half hours. or until the beef is tender. In a small bowl, combine water and cornstarch; stir in beef mixture. Bake for another 15 minutes or until sauce thickens. Per serving: cal 180, fat 4 g, fat sat 1g, chol 60 mg, turf 440 mg, carbohydrates 8 g, fib 1 g, prot 27 g

Swiss Steak
Makes 6 servings

1 1/2 lbs boneless boneless beef steak, about 3/4" thick
1/2 teaspoon.
6 to 8 new potatoes, cut into fourth
1 1/2 cups carrots, cut by baby
1 med. onion, sliced
1 can (14 1/2 oz) diced tomatoes with basil,
garlic and oregano, 12 oz unsplugged jar of
chopped fresh chopped beef sauce, if
desired

Remove excess beef. Cut beef into 6pc of serving. Spray the 12-inch pan with cooking spray; heat over low heat. Sprinkle beef with seasoned salt. Cook the beef in the pan for about 8 minutes, turning once, until golden. Place potatoes, carrots, beef and onion in a slow cookery for 3 1/2 to 6 qt. Mix tomatoes and sauce; spoon on beef and vegetables.

Cover and cook on LOW 7-9 hours. or until the beef and vegetables are tender. Sprinkle with parsley.

Per serving: cal 275, 5g fat, 2g sat fat, sat 60mg chol, 600mg turf, 34g carbohydrates, 4g fibre, prot 28g

Tarragona-Mustard Turkey with Fettuccine
Makes 4-6 servings

1 lb boneless, skinless turkey breast
2 leeks
2 celery stalks, chopped
1 tbsp chopped fresh tarragon
2 tsp Dijon mustard
1 tbsp fresh lemon juice
1 tbsp brown sugar
1 tsp instant chicken broth granules 1/4 tsp
salt
1/8 tsp ground black pepper 2
tbsp Cornstarch
2 tbsp cold water
6 to 8 oz fettucine or medication. masta shells

Cut the turkey into thin strips, about 1 x 1/4". Cut leeks; halve lengthwise. Rinse and slice. Mix turkey and leeks in a slow 3 1/2 qt pane with celery. In a small bowl, combine tarragon, lemon juice, mustard, brown sugar, broth granules, salt and pepper. Pour over turkey. Cover and cook on LOW 4 1/2 to 5 hours. or until turkey and vegetables are tender. Turn the control to HIGH. Dissolve cornstarch in a small bowl. Stir the cooking juices into a slow cooker. Cover and cook on HIGH for 20-30 min. or until thickened. Cook pasta in pkg directions. and drain. Pour turkey mixture over cooked pasta.

Per serving: cal 271, carb 48g, pro 41g, fat 1g, sat fat 0g, chol 90mg, turf 280mg

Teriyaki Steak
6 portions

1 LB Flank Steak
1/4 C Soy Sauce
1C pineapple pieces in juice - Drained, 1/4 cup reserved juice 1 Tsp.
Ginger Root - grated
1 tbsp sugar
1 tbsp oil
2 Crushed garlic clove
3 Tbs. Cornstarch
3 Tbs. Eau

Cut the meat into 1/8-inch slices and place in a low slow cooker. In a small bowl, combine soy sauce, reserved pineapple juice, ginger, sugar oil and garlic. Pour the sauce mixture over the meat. Cover and cook on LOW 6 to 7 hours. Turn the control to HIGH. Stir in pineapple. Combine cornstarch and water in a small bowl; add to the stove. Cook, stirring, until slightly thickened. Serve on rice...........................

Per serving (excluding unknown items): 210 calories; 10g fat (44.0% calories from fat); 15g protein; 14g carbohydrates; dietary fibre trace; 39mg cholesterol; 740mg sodium.

Texas Chili
Makes 6 servings (1 2/3 cups)

1 1/2 lbs round beef steak, decked out, cut into 3/4-inch cubes 1
small onion, finely chopped
2 garlic cloves, finely chopped
1 (28 oz) can make diced tomatoes, not
1 (8 oz) tomato sauce
1 (15.5 oz or 16 oz) pintobeans, unsplunted 1 (4.5 oz)
can chopped green peppers
3 tsp chili powder
1 tsp Cumin

Toppings: (Not included in analysis)
Sour cream, shredded cheddar cheese, sliced green onions

In the 4 to 6 qt slow cooker, combine all the chili ingredients; mix well. Cover; cook on LOW for 8-10 hours. To serve, lay the chilli in bowls. Add toppings, if desired.

Per serving: cal 330, fat 10g, fat sat 5g, chol 75mg, carbohydrates 27g, fib 7g, prot 32g

Tex-Mex Bean Stew with cornmeal dumplings

1 15 oz can red beans, rinsed and drained 1 15 oz can black
beans rinsed and drained
3 cups water
1 14 1/2 oz Mexican-style simmered tomatoes
1 10 oz package frozen whole corn, thawed 2 medium
carrots, sliced (1 cup)
1 large onion, chopped (1 cup)
1 4 oz chopped green peppers
2 tsp chicken broth granules
1 to 2 tsp chili powder
2 garlic cloves, chopped 1/3
cup all-purpose flour 1/4
cup yellow cornmeal 1 tsp
Salt dash baking powder
Dash pepper
1 egg white, beaten
2 Tbs. Lait
1 Tbs. cooking oil

In 3-1/1/2 or 4-quarter electric dishes, combine canned beans, water, tomatoes, corn, carrots, onion, non brontan peppers,,   broth granules, chili powder and garlic. Cover and cook over low heat for 10 to 12 hours or set at high temperature for 4 to 5 hours.

For the meatballs, in a small mixing bowl, combine flour, cornmeal, baking powder, salt and pepper. In another small mixing bowl, combine egg white, milk and cooking oil. Add the white egg mixture to the flour mixture; stir with a fork just until combined. If the stew is cooked over low heat, turn the dishtop in a high heat setting. Place the meatball mixture in 8 teaspoons rounded at the top of the stew.

Cover; cook for another 30 minutes (do not lift the lid).

Makes 4 servings.
(Calories 391, Fat 6g, Fibre 12g)

Tex-Mex Chicken 'N' Rice

Service size: 8

2 cups converted, uncooked rice; Uncle Ben
28 ounces diced tomatoes, Hunt's
6 ounces tomato paste
3 cups hot water
1 packing taco seasoning mixture
1 pound boneless, skinless chicken breast -- cut into 1/2-inch cubes 2
medium onions -- chopped
1 medium green pepper -- chopped
4 ounces green peppers -- diced
3/4 teaspoon garlic pepper

In a slow cooker, combine all ingredients except chillies and garlic pepper. Cover and cook over low heat for 4 to 4 and a half hours or until rice is tender and chicken is white everywhere; don't overcook or the rice will be soft. Stir in chillies and peppers with garlic. Serve immediately.

Calories: 174.3 Grams of fat: 1.1 Grams of fiber: 3.0

Tex-Mex Turkey Envelope

Donne 16 wraps

2 lbs turkey breast fillets 1/4
teaspoon seasoned salt
1/4 teaspoon pepper
1 m onion, chopped (1/2 cup) 1/3
cup water
2 envelopes (1 1/4 oz each) taco seasoning mixture
16 flour tortillas (8-10" in diameter)
2 cups of pcs the size of a mouthful. Lettuce
2 cups grated cheddar cheese (8 oz)

Place turkey in 3 1/2-4 qt. Slow cooker. Sprinkle with seasoned salt and pepper. Add onion and water. Cover and cook on LOW 6-7 hours. or until the turkey juice is no longer pink when the thickest parts centres are cut. Remove turkey from slow cooker. Shred turkey, using 2 forks. Measure the fluid from the slow cooker; add enough water to the liquid to measure 2 cups. Mix the seasoning mixtures (dry) and the liquid mixture in a slow cooker. Stir in grated turkey. Cover and cook on LOW 1 hour. Pour about 1/4 cup of turkey into the centre of each tortilla; garnish with lettuce and cheese. Roll tortillas.

By wrapping. cal 260,8g fat, 4g sat fat, 50mg chol, 540mg turf, carb 28g, 2g fibre, prot 22g

Three Pepper Steak

Makes 5-6 servings

1 (1 to 1 1/4 lbs) beef belly steak
1 yellow pepper
1 green pepper 1/4
teaspoon salt
1/2 teaspoon red pepper flakes
3 green onions, some of which are high, chopped
2 tbsp soy sauce
Two med. tomatoes, chopped

Cut all the visible fat from the steak. Place steak in 3 1/2 qt slow cooker. Remove stems and seeds from yellow and green peppers; cut into strips. Arrange peppers on steak. Sprinkle with salt. Garnish with red pepper flakes, green onions, soy sauce and tomatoes. Cover and cook on lOW 6-7 hours. or until the steak is tender.

Per serving: cal 163, carb 5g, prot 21g, 7g fat, sat 3g fat, chol 45mg, turf 590mg

Tomato-Tortilla soup

Makes 6 servings

4 cups crushed tomatoes
1 1/4 cups vegetable stock
2 qniles, finely chopped
3 garlic cloves, finely chopped
2 dried cayenne peppers, chopped or 2 tsp crushed red pepper flakes 1 tbsp
dried parsley
6 corn tortillas, cut into 3/4-inch strips
1 cup (4 oz) grated Monterey Jack cheese

Mix the first 6 ingredients in the slow cooker. Cover and cook on LOW 7-9 hours. or on HIGH 3 1/2 to 5 hours. Place tortillas on baking sheet and mix with olive oil spray. Grill until crisp and golden, about 5 min.

Divide the soup among 6 bowls and top each serving with tortilla strips and cheese.

Per serving: 210 cal, 6.6 g fat, 3.7 g sat fat, 17 mg chol, 421 mg turf, 3.7 g fib

Touch of oriental chicken

6 whole chicken thighs - not quarter leg 1/2
cup soy sauce
1/4 cup light brown sugar 2
garlic cloves -- chopped 1 8 oz
tomato sauce

Remove skin from chicken. Use a paper towel to make this slippery task easier. He grabs the chicken like magic! Put the chicken in a slow cooker. In a medium bowl, combine soy sauce, brown sugar, garlic and tomato sauce and mix well. Pour sauce over chicken. Cover and cook over low heat for about 6 to 8 hours or until chicken is tender. Serve with rice. Sometimes I like to use 12 boneless thighs and break it into bite-sized pieces when they are tender, then throw in a bag of frozen oriental vegetables. You can thicken the sauce with a little cornstarch, if desired. Yield: 6 - 8 servings This gel well.

Tuna noodle casserole

4 portions

2 cans celery soup 1/3 cup dry
sherry
2/3 cup skimmed milk
2 tablespoons parsley flakes
10 ounces frozen peas
2 can tuna - drained
10 ounces egg noodles -- cooked (no yolk)
2 tablespoons light margarine
1 Dash curry powder -- (optional)

In a large bowl, carefully mix soup, sherry, milk, parsley flakes, vegetables and tuna. Stir in noodles. Pour into greased crock-pot. Sprinkle with butter or margarine. Cover and cook over low heat for 7 to 9 hours. (Cook the noodles untiltender.)

Turkey Crock Casserole

1 1/2 cups diced (8 ounces) cooked turkey breast
10 slices of reduced-calorie bread, processed into soft crumbs
3/4 cup celery
1/4 cup chopped onion
2 cups Campbell's Healthy Request chicken broth (16 ounces can) 3
tablespoons all-purpose flour
1/2 teaspoon poultry seasoning 1/4
teaspoon black pepper
1 teaspoon dried parsley flakes

In a slow cooker container, combine turkey, breadcrumbs, celery and onion. In a covered jar, combine chicken broth and flour. Shake well. Pour the mixture into a medium saucepan sprayed with a butter-flavoured cooking spray. Cook over medium heat, stirring often, until mixture thickens. Stir in poultry seasoning, black pepper and parsley flakes. Pour broth mixture over turkey mixture. Mix well to combine. Cover and cook over low heat for 6 to 8 hours.

Serves 6 (1 cup). Each serving is equivalent to: 145 calories, 1 gram of fat, 18 grams of protein, 16 grams of carbohydrates, 343 milligrams of sodium and 1 gram of fiber. Tip: 1. If you don't have leftovers, buy a piece of cooked turkey breast from your local deli.

Turkey-Tomato soup

1 pound turkey legs, boneless, peeled -- cut into 1" (2" (2 medium) 2 small red
potatoes -- cubed (or white)
1 3/4 cups reduced-sodium, fat-free chicken broth 1 1/2
cups frozen corn
1 cup chopped onion
1 cup water
8 ounces salted tomato sauce without salt -- (1 can)
1/4 cup tomato paste
2 tablespoons Dijon mustard
1 teaspoon hot pepper sauce 1/2
teaspoon sugar
1/2 teaspoon garlic powder
1/4 cup finely chopped fresh parsley

In a slow cooker, combine all ingredients except parsley. Cover and cook on LOW 9 to 10 hours. Stir in parsley; Serve.
Makes 6 servings. Per serving: 223 calories; 8g fat; 52g protein; 22g Carbohydrates; 3g dietary fibre; 38mg cholesterol; 415mg sodium. Service Ideas: Serve this soup with thick sliced whole grain bread for a nutritious and hearty weekday dinner.

Tuscan pasta

1 pound boneless skinless chicken breasts, cut into 1 inch 1 can (15
1/2 ounces) red beans, rinsed and drained 1 can (15 oz
each)Italian-style simmered tomatoes
1 jar (4 1/2oz) sliced mushrooms, drained
1 med. green pepper, chopped 1/2 cup
onion, chopped
1/2 cup celery, chopped 4
cloves garlic, chopped 1 cup
water
1 tsp dried Italian seasoning
6 oz thin spaghetti, halved

Place all ingredients except spaghetti in slow cooker. Cover and cook on LOW for 4 hours or until vegetables are tender. Turn to HIGH. Stir in spaghetti; Cover. Stir again after 10 minutes. Cover and cook for 45 minutes or until pasta is tender. Garnish with basil and pepper strips, if desired.

Cal per serving: 272 Fat 2g   dietary fibre: 6gOF SERVES8

Vegetable Medley

4 cups peeled potatoes, diced
1 1/2 cups frozen whole corn
4 medium tomatoes, seeded and diced
1 cup carrots, sliced 1/2
chopped onion 3/4
teaspoon salt 1/2
teaspoon sugar

1/2 teaspoon dill disedure
1/8 teaspoon pepper

Mix all ingredients in a slow cooker. **Cover and** cook over low heat for **5 to 6 hours or until vegetables are tender. Yield 8 (1 cup each)** serving per serving Calories: 116 Fat: 1g (sat: trace) Fibre: 4g Chol:0 Sod:: 243mg Carb:27g Prot::3g

Vegetarian marine bean soup

16 ounces of sea beans -- rinsed
8 cups water
1 cup carrots -- finely chopped
1 cup celery -- finely chopped and leaves
1/2 cup onion -- finely chopped
1 cup tomato vegetable cocktail juice
1 tablespoon chicken-flavoured instant broth 1/8
teaspoon crushed red pepper flakes

In a large saucepan or Oven, combine beans and water. Bring to a boil. Boil for 30 minutes; remove from the heat. Leave to rest for 1-1/2 hours or until beans are tender. In slow cooker, combine beans (and water) and all remaining ingredients; mix well. Cover and cook at low setting for 6 to 8 hours or until beans and vegetables are very tender.

8 servings (1 cup). Per serving: 211 calories; 1 g fat; 13g protein; 39g carbohydrates; 15g dietary fibre; cholesterol trace; 284mg sodium.

White bean pepper and green pepper soup

30 ounces large, canned northern beans -- (2 - 15 oz) rinsed and drained 1 cup finely
chopped yellow onion
4 1/2 ounces diced green peppers -- (1 can)
1 teaspoon ground cumin - 1/2
teaspoon garlic powder
14 1/2 ounces fat-free chicken broth -- (1 can) 1/4
cup chopped fresh coriander leaves
1 tablespoon extra virgin olive oil 1/3
cup extra virgin sour cream

Combine beans, onion, chillies, 1/2 teaspoon cumin and garlic powder in a slow cooker. Cook on LOW 8 hours or on HIGH 4 hours. Stir in coriander, olive oil and remaining one to second teaspoon of cumin. Garnish with sour cream, if desired. Makes 5 servings.

Per serving: 280 calories; 7g fat; 17g protein; 42g carbohydrates; 9g dietary fibre; 7mg Cholesterol; 222mg sodium.

White Chile

1 pound dried northern beans, rinsed and sorted
4 cups chicken broth
2 cups chopped onions
3 garlic cloves, finely chopped
2 teaspoons ground cumin
1-1/2 teaspoon dried oregano
1 teaspoon ground coriander 1/8
teaspoon ground cloves 1/8
teaspoon cayenne pepper
1 can (4 oz) chopped green peppers
1/2 pound boneless skinless chicken breasts, toasted and cubed 1
teaspoon salt

Place beans in a soup kettle or Oven in the Netherlands; add 2-inch water to cover. Bring to a boil. Boil for 2 minutes. Remove from heat; cover and let stand for 1 hour. Drain and rinse the beans, throwing in the liquid. Put the beans in a slow cooker. Add broth, onions, garlic and seasonings. Cover and cook over low heat for 7 to 8 hours or until beans are almost tender. Add chillies, chicken and salt; cover and cook for 1 hour or until beans are tender. Serve with cheese if desired.

6 servings (1-1/3 cups) 384 calories; 5 grams of fat; 16 grams of fiber

Vienna bean pot

20 ounces (2 16oz)   large northern beans rinsed and drained 1 3/4 cups (a
15 oz) oz) Hunting tomato sauce
2 tbsp Twin I tbs brown
sugar. mustard prepared a
teaspoon of dried parsley
12 oz Healthy Choice 97% fat-free frankfurters diced 1/2
cup chopped onion

In a slow cooker container, combine large Nordic beans, tomato sauce, brown sugar twin, mustard and parsley flakes. Add the frankfurters and onion. Mix well to combine. Cover and cook on LOW for 6-8 hours. Mix well before serving.

For 6 (1 cup) Each serving is equivalent to: 193 Calories I gm fat, 16 gm pr,,30 gm ca,978 mg. So 70 mg Cl 7 gm Fi